The Nutritional Value of

Indigenous Wild Plants:

An Annotated Bibliography

The Nutritional Value of

Indigenous Wild Plants:

An Annotated Bibliography

by

John R. K. Robson

and

Joel N. Elias

The Whitston Publishing Company
Troy, New York
1978

TABLE OF CONTENTS

INTRODUCTION

The Malthusian axiom, that population growth will rapidly outstrip food supplies and thereby lead to biological catastrophe, has proven correct for many countries in recent years. Because the total quantity of land suitable for western agriculture is indeed limited, research efforts have largely focused on the development of high-yielding crop varieties which, in addition, require optimal growing conditions to achieve maximum yields. To create these conditions has necessitated great investment of energy in the form of fuel, fertilizers and pesticides, not the mention the energy spent in the development, production and shipment of complicated machinery to the remotest parts of the globe.

Yet, even the Green Revolution has been unable to alleviate world hunger, and population growth in the developing countries has continued to accelerate despite impressive agricultural gains.

Advocates of the Third World have become increasingly critical of the uses to which the developed nations have committed significant portions of the world's limited food supply. They cite the wastefulness and overnutrition so prevalent among affluent populations while others starve. Most of all, they point to the wasteful conversion of important protein foods into animal products whereby as much as seven to ten pounds of grain is used to produce but a single pound of beef. This grain could have been used more effectively to feed people. This extravagance clearly indicates the need for a more equitable distribution of food as well as a reexamination of all food materials.

In present systems of agriculture there are inherent problems which increasingly focus on techniques of mechanized farming. Monoculture, the raising of but one type of crop on a parcel of land, so simplifies the ecosystem on that land that serious imbalances in the system are likely to occur. Crop rotation and replacement of primary soil nutrients by fertilizers attempt to compensate for these imbalances, but they may prove inadequate over the long run. Similarly, the use of pesticides to prevent the widespread depredation to which such overly-simplified systems are vulnerable is again a costly and inadequate solution.

Millions of dollars have been spent to adapt what are primarily temperate climate crops, such as wheat and maize, to regions of the world where they are illsuited to grow. It is noteworthy that virtually all of the efforts to improve man's food supply have focused on improving cultigens which were already the mainstay of civilizations countless centuries ago. Corn, beans, wheat, and rice—to name just a few—were all indentified and domesticated by aboriginal populations having no techniques at their disposal other than those of primitive agriculture and artificial selection. Trial and error over generations produced results. These simple methods today can be supplemented or replaced by the sciences of toxicology, genetics, agriculture and nutrition. Forty years ago Vavilov started to track down the wild varieties of the many cultigens in an attempt to collect sufficient germplasm to produce new varieties possessing hybrid qualities derived from their wild relatives.

Yet, it still remains for plant scientists to devote themselves seriously to the question of whether there are other, less well-known cultigens (such as *Iva annua, Chenopodium* spp., *Amaranthus* spp., etc.) which with our more sophisticated techniques of plant science could be bred to a level of productivity comparable to the major, present-day crops. The benefits from such an undertaking would be two-fold. First, there is much land in the world unsuited to crop production. This is especially true for the present assortment of high-yield cultigens. Reasons for this include problems of soil, climate and the vulnerability of known crops to endemic pest infestations. But, there are plants which do survive and prosper within these areas, and they might be identified, improved and used as additional food sources. Furthermore, the diversification of crop types would increase the likelihood of developing heterocultural systems, and this could lead to higher nutrient yields on a year-round basis with lowered energy costs. This would be specially valuable for tropical areas where duplication of the natural plant succession using food-producing herbs, shrubs, and trees would help to reduce damage to already marginally fertile soil types.

But, in addition to the need to bring new genera under cultivation in order to expand food production to environments presently inaccessible to our food crops, we must also consider the need for alternative food resources for livestock.

The fact that ruminants are capable of digesting and utilizing plant materials in ways which humans cannot should lead us to seek energy and protein-rich animal foods which would take livestock out of competition with humans by giving them foods which cannot be consumed by humans. For example, the inner bark of many trees is a relatively rich source of amino acids. One might question whether this by-product of the lumber industry could be refined and utilized in some way as a potential feed for herbivorous animals. Others have suggested similar uses for the leaf protein present in many of the aquatic plants that often choke our inland waterways.

By expanding the range of environments suitable for agriculture and by finding alternative feeds for livestock, we might greatly increase the food supply of humans. At the same time efforts must be made to reduce the total input of chemical energy needed for food production.

In our effort to learn more of the food potential of indigenous foods we were frustrated in our efforts to quickly locate literature containing information on their nutrient content. Communication with librarians and specialists in various scientific fields indicated that there was no easy way to locate such material short of searching for it journal by journal. Much information existed, it was generally agreed, but no one knew exactly where to find it. It was subsequently decided to undertake a literature search and make the results available to others who might find such an annotated bibliography useful.

The resulting bibliography is the product of more than a year's work. It is not all-inclusive, nor does it include works more recent than 1972 or 1973. What it does do is to bring together the bulk of the important literature on the subject and presents that literature in a manner that permits one to locate works according to the genera and/or species of interest and indicates the type of analyses reported. In this way it may be possible to gain access to more recent literature in the field.

Although many of the genera reported on are not native to North America, it was decided that they be included as part of the modern flora of that region. It was also realized at the outset of the study that, were we to have attempted to annotate all articles reporting nutrient analyses of "wild" plants regardless of the region of the world from which those plants came, the bibliography might have taken years to compile. Lacking time, personnel and funds, we thus restricted ourselves to the North American continent and left other regions for future volumes.

It is hoped that this work will save others time in searching the literature and will thereby make research into the area of alternative foods and feedstuffs more attractive.

At this time we would like to acknowledge the Rodale Press and the University of Michigan Human Nutrition Program without whose generous support and facilities this project could not have been completed. We also wish to express thanks to the clerical staff of the Human Nutrition Program, especially Mrs. Geraldine Pease who typed the manuscript, for their help and moral support over the many months of work.

A

1. Adams, Wm. E., M. Stelly, R. A. McCreery, H. D. Morris and Charles B. Elkins, Jr.

    1966 Protein, P, and K composition of coastal bermuda-grass and crimson clover. *J. Range Mgmt.* 19(5):301-305.

    Species: *Cynodon dactylon* (L.) Pers.; *Trifolium incarnatum.*

2. Adrian, J., P. Lunven and E. Carnovale

    1969 L'alpiste. I. L'alpiste des oiseaux (*Phalaris canariensis* L.). Une source exceptionelle de tryptophane. (Phalaris I. Canary grass (*Phalaris canariensis* L.), an exceptional source of tryptophan.) *Ann. Nutrition Aliment.* 23:299-312, in French.

    Nutr. Abstr., 1970, 40:807.

    Proximate and amino acid analyses of *P. canariensis* L. and *P. arundinacea* (reed canary grass from Canada.)

3. Akeson, W. R. and M. A. Stahmann

    1965 Nutritive value of leaf protein concentrate, an *in vitro* digestion study. *J. Agric. Food Chem.* 13:145-148.

    Nutr. Abstr., 35:5525.

Akeson, W. R. and M. A. Stahmann (cont.)

Analysis of release of 16 amino acids with treatment by *in vitro* sequential pepsin and pancreatin hydrolysis; estimates of biological value of proteins.

Species: *Chenopodium, Nasturtium,* rye grass, clover, and various cultigens analyzed.

4.   Aldous, Shaler E.

1952   Deer browse clipping study in the lake states region. *J. Wildl. Mgmt.* 16(3):401-409.

Percent H_2O tabulated for young shoots with the exception of *Thuja.*

Species: *Thuja occidentalis, Acer spicatum, Betula alba* var. *papyrifera, Sorbus americanus, Cornus stolonifera, Prunus pennsylvanica, Sambucus racemosa, Salix* sp., *Fraxinus nigra.*

5.   Alkon, Philip U.

1961   Nutritional and acceptability values of hardwood slash as winter deer browse. *J. Wildl. Mgmt.* 25(1):77-81.

Proximate analyses on twigs collected from September through March.

Species: *Acer rubrum, A. saccharum, Betula papyrifera.*

6.   Alway, F. J., T. E. Maki and W. J. Methley

1934   Composition of the leaves of some forest trees. *Am. Soil Assn. Bull.* No. 15, p. 87.

June-September collections percent ash, CaO, MgO, P_2O_5 and N.

6

Alway, F. J., T. E. Maki and W. J. Methley (cont.)

Species: 9 forest species: 2 maple species, 3 oak species, green ash, boxelder, American elm and basswood.

7. Ames. S. R.

1971 Determination of vitamin E in foods and feeds—a collaborative study. *J. Assn. Official Analytical Chem.* 54(1): 1-12.

Nutr. Abstr., 42:5448.

8. Andreasi, F., F. Prada, C. X. Mendonca, Jr. and J. S. M. Veiga

1969 Survey of chemical composition of forage plants in defined areas of the state of Sao Paulo. *Rev. Fac. Med. Vet. Sao Paulo* 8(1):159-175. Portuguese: English Summary.

Nutr. Abstr. 42:378.

9. Appelqvist, L. A.

1968 Lipids in Cruciferae: I. Fatty acid composition in seeds of some Svalof varieties and strains of rape, turnip rape, white mustard and false flax. *Acta Agric. Scand.* 18:3-21.

Nutr. Abstr. 39:325.

10. —.

1970 Lipids in Cruciferae: VI. The fatty acid composition of seeds of some cultivated *Brassica* species and of *Sinapis alba* L. *Fette: Seifen: Anstrichmittel,* 72:783-792.

Nutr. Abstr. 41:2399.

Appelqvist, L. A. (cont.)

> Species: *Brassica campestris, B. carinata, B. juncea, B. napus, B. nigra, B. oleracea,* and *Sinapis alba.*

11. Archibald, J. G., E. Bennet and W. S. Ritchie

> 1943 The composition and palatability of some common grasses. *J. Agr. Res.* 66:341-347.
>
> Proximate contents, Mg, and Vitamin A (in I.U.) for 7 species of grasses. Also, proximate contents of 2 sp. of clover.
>
> Species: *Poa pratensis, Dactylis glomerata, Agrostis alba, Agrostis capillaris, Phleum pratense, Festuca ovina, Anthoxanthum odoratum, Trifolium repens.*

12. Armsby, Henry Prentiss

> 1888 Nutritive value of pasture grass. Pa. Agr. Exp. Sta. *Ann. Rept.* pp. 60-77.

13. Atkeson, F. W., W. J. Peterson and A. E. Aldous

> 1937 Observations on the carotene content of some typical pasture plants. *J. Dairy Sci.* 20:557-562.
>
> Species: *Andropogon furcatus, A. scoparius, Buchloë dactyloides.*

14. Atwood, Earl L.

> 1948 A nutritional knowledge shortcut. *J. Wildl. Mgmt.* 12(1): 1-8.
>
> Proximate composition of deer foods.

Atwood, Earl L. (cont.)

Species: *Ulmus americana*, leaves, shoots, twigs; *Quercus vellutina*, acorns; *Q. alba*, leaves, twigs; *Cornus racemosa*, shoots; *C. stolonifera*, leaves, shoots; *Carya ovata*, leaves; *Acer saccharinum*, leaves, shoots; *A. saccharum*, leaves, twigs; *Corylus americana*, shoots; *Rubus occidentalis*, leaves; *Solidago hispida*, leaves; *Rhus glabra*, leaves, fruit, canes; *Vitis bicolor*, leaves, tendrils.

15. Austin, F. L. and I. A. Wolff

1968 Sinapine and related esters in seed meal of *Crambe abyssinica. J. Agr. Food Chem.* 16(1):132-135.

16. Averill, H. P. and C. G. Averill

1962 Chemical constituents of nuts. *J. Am. Chem. Soc.* 48: 724-728.

17. Aylward, F.

1953 The indigenous foods of Mexico and Central America. Symposium of The Nutrition Society on Unusual Foods for Human Consumption, 18, October, 1952. *Proceedings of the Nutrition Society* 12(1):48-58.

Good bibliography; review of work of Robert Harris analyses of some 250 varieties of food for moisture, crude fibre, ether extract, N, P, Ca, *Fe*, ascorbic acid, thiamine, ribovlavin, niacin, and Vitamin A (as carotene).

B

18. Bagby, M. O. and C. R. Smith, Jr.

    1967 Asymmetric triglycerides from *Impatiens edgeworthii* seed
          oil. *Biochem. Biophys. Acta.* 137(3):475-477.

19. Bagby, M. O., C. R. Smith, Jr. and I. A. Wolff

    1964 A naturally occurring allenic acid from *Leonotis nepetae-
          folia* seed oil. *Chem. Ind.* (London) 45:1861-1862.

20. —

    1965 Labellenic acid. A new allenic acid from *Leonotis nepet-
          aefolia* seed oil. *J. Org. Chem.* 30(12):4227-4229.

21. —.

    1966 Stereochemistry of d-parinaric acid from *Impatiens edge-
          worthii* seed oil. *Lipids* 1(4):263-267.

22. Bagby, M. O., C. R. Smith, Jr., K. L. Mikolajczak and I. A.
     Wolff

    1962 *Thalictrum polycarpum* fatty acids—a new class of fatty
          acids from vegetable seed oils. *Biochemistry* 1(4):632-
          639.

23. Bagby, M. O., C. R. Smith, Jr., T. K. Miwa, R. L. Lohmar
     and I. A. Wolff

    1961 A unique fatty acid from *Limnanthes douglasii* seed oil:
          The C_{22} diene. *J. Org. Chem.* 26(4):1261-1265.

24. Bagby, M. O., W. O. Seigl and I. A. Wolff

    1965 A new acid from *Calea urticaefolia* seed oil: *Trans-3, Cis-9, Cis-12-octadecatrienoic acid. J. Amer. Oil Chemists' Soc.* 42(1):50-53.

25. Bailey, E. M.

    1927 The thirty-first report on food products and the nineteenth report on drug products, 1926. Part II, food and drug inspection. Conn. Agr. Exp. Sta. *Bulletin*, No. 287, pp. 339-390, New Haven.

    Proximate analysis of acorns.

26. —.

    1942 Commercial feeding stuffs. Report on inspection, 1941. Conn. Agr. Exp. Sta. *Bulletin,* No. 459, pp. 329-422, New Haven.

    Proximate analyses of native grains, seeds and berries.

27. —.

    1943 Commercial feeding stuffs. Report on inspection, 1942. Conn. Agr. Exp. Sta. *Bulletin,* No. 473, pp. 317-434, New Haven.

    Proximate analyses of native fruits, seeds and berries.

28. —.

    1945 Commercial feeding stuffs. Report on inspection, 1944. Conn. Agr. Exp. Sta. *Bulletin,* No. 486, pp. 165-260, New Haven.

    Proximate analyses of native grains, seeds and berries.

29. Bailey, James A.

　　1967　Sampling deer browse for crude protein. *J. Wildl. Mgmt.*
　　　　　31(3):437-442.

　　　　　Species: *Viburnum alnifolium.*

30. —.

　　1969　Exploratory study of nutrition of young cottontails.
　　　　　J. Wildl. Mgmt. 33(2):346-353.

　　　　　Seasonal analysis dry matter percent, protein percent,
　　　　　Energy Kcal/g.

　　　　　Species: *Poa* sp., *Dactylis glomerata, Phleum pratense,
　　　　　Medicago sativa, Trifolium pratense, Melilotus* sp., *Cichor-
　　　　　ium intybus, Lactuca scariola, Plantago rugelii, Ambrosia
　　　　　trifida, Aster pilosus, Polygonum* sp., *Amaranthus retro-
　　　　　flexus, Chenopodium album.*

31. Bailey, L. F.

　　1948　Leaf oils from Tennessee Valley conifers. *J. For.* 46:882-
　　　　　889.

　　　　　Oil yield, specific gravity and principal components. (20
　　　　　refs.)

　　　　　Summary of the literature; 26 species (leaves and small
　　　　　twigs) reported.

32. Banthorpe, D. V. et al.

　　1973　Monoterpene patterns in *Juniperus* and *Thuja* species.
　　　　　Planta Med. 23:64-69.

33. Bard, G. E.

   1946   The mineral nutrient content of the foliage of forest trees on three soil types of varying limestone content. *Proc. Soil Sci. Soc. of Amer.* 10:419-422.

   Twenty-five species of trees: foliar contents of Ca, P, N, and K reported.

   Soil types: Honeoye, Lansing and Bath silt loams.

34. Barnes, R. L.

   1962   Glutamine synthesis and translocation in pine. *Plant Physiol.* 37:323-326.

35. —.

   1963   Nitrogen transport in the xylem of trees. *J. For.* 61:50-51.

36. Barnes, R. L. and G. W. Bengtson

   1968   Effects of fertilization, irrigation and cover cropping flowering and on nitrogen and soluble sugar composition of slash pine. *For. Sci.* 14(2):172-180.

   Twigs (first plush) amino acid tot. (umoles/g fresh wt.) arginine, tot. soluble sugars (mg/g fresh wt.), reducing sugar moisture tot. N., fresh wt.; needles: tot. N.

   Clonal differences examined.

   Pinus elliottii Engelm.

37. Barnes, Robert L.

   1963   Organic nitrogen compounds in the tree xylem sap. *For.*

Barnes, Robert L. (cont.)

Sci. 9(1):98-102.

1) Percent distribution of N among free amino acids found in xylem sap of 7 species of pine.

2) Amino acids and ureides found in saps of 60 species studied.

3) Classification of 60 species according to the main amino acid or ureide found in the xylem sap.

4) Classification of 28 families according to the main amino acid or ureide found in the sap of the species studied.

38. Barr, C. G.

1942 Reserve foods in the roots of whiteweed (*Cardaria Draba var. repens*). *J. Agr. Res.* 64(12):725-740.

Seasonal trends in the carbohydrate and nitrogen content (percent) of whiteweed roots in the first—and second—foot levels of undisturbed and cultivated plants are calculated and plotted against date of sampling on a fresh-wt. basis. The effect of sodium chlorate and cultivation on the carbohydrate content of whiteweed roots is also analyzed.

39. Barshad, Isaac

1948 Molybdenum content of pasture plants in relation to toxicity to cattle. *Soil Sci.* 66:187-195.

For legumes and grasses—1) Mo in ppm for both soil and 22 species of pasture N plant, 2) Mo content of 2 varieties of *Lotus corniculatus* growing in the same pot, 3) Effect of season on Mo content of plants (leaves and stems of 8 species), 4) Mo content of leaves in relation to age (3

Barshad, Isaac (cont.)

species), legumes contain higher quantities of Mo than
non-leguminous plants because N fixing bacteria require
Mo.

40. —.

1951   Factors affecting the molybdenum content of pasture
plants I. Nature of soil molybdenum, growth of plants,
and soil pH. *Soil Sci.* 71(4):297-314.

Analyses of leaves, stem, seed and fruit of 20 species
grown in the loam soil; and 15 species grown in 6 soil
types compared.

Concentration of (Mo) in plants increases with age and is
directly related to water soluble Mo in soil (pH 4.7-7.5).
Mo uptake suppressed at pH > 7.5.

41. Barua, J., R. Valdivia, V. Kato, L. Campos and J. de Soko

1967   Analysis of forages and concentrates. *Lab. Biochem.
Animal Nutri.*, Vet. Fac., Univ. Nac Mayor de San Marcos,
July, 1967, p. 7, mimeographed.

Nutr. Abstr., 38:6780.

Proximate composition and Ca, P and Mg contents tabulated for 18 green forage and silage species and 40 pasture
species.

42. Bates, T. E.

1971   Factors affecting critical nutrient concentrations in plants
and their evaluation: a review. *Soil Sci.* 112(2):116-130.

43. Beauchamp, E. G., T. H. Lane, R. B. Carson and M. Hidiroglou

    1969 A note on selenium contents of two leguminous forage species collected in Ontario and the possible incidence of selenium-responsive diseases. *Canad. Vet. J.* 10:193-194.

    Nutr. Abstr., 40:2557.

    Analysis of 117 samples of lucerne (*Medicago sativa*) and 4 samples of birdsfoot trefoil: range of Se concentration: lucerne 99 samples 0.030-0.089 ppm (9 samples < .03 ppm) and trefoil 0.02-0.039 ppm.

44. Beath, D. A. and J. W. Hamilton

    1952 Chemical composition of Wyoming forage plants. Wyo. Agr. Exp. Sta. *Bulletin*, 311, 40 pp.

45. Beck, John R. and D. O. Beck

    1955 A method for nutritional evaluation of wildlife foods. *J. Wildl. Mgmt.* 19(2):198-205.

    Proximate and mineral analyses of 39 wild turkey foods. (Ca, Zn, Mg, P, Fe) reported.

46. Beeson, K. C.

    1946 The effect of mineral supply on the mineral concentration and nutritional quality of plants. *Bot. Rev.* 12:424-455.

    Review of literature on fertilization trials and effects of micronutrients on the mineral composition of plants (124 refs.).

47. —.

   1959   Plant and soil analysis in the evaluation of micronutrient
          element status.   Duke Univ. School Forestry *Bulletin,*
          15:71-80.

          Discussion of the relationship between soils and the mi-
          cronutrient uptake in plants (24 refs.).

48. Beeson, K. C. and H. A. MacDonald

   1951   Absorption of mineral elements by forge plants: III. The
          relation of stage of growth to the micronutrient element
          content of timothy and some legumes. *Agron. J.* 43:589-
          593.

          Plotted relation of stage of growth to the contents of Co,
          Cu, Fe and Mn (ppm) in alfalfa, ladino clover, birdsfoot
          trefoil and timothy hay.

49. Bell, E. A.

   1960   Canavanine in the Leguminosae. *Biochem. J.* 75:618.

          Report on Canavanine in seeds of the Leguminosae fami-
          ly.   Method and results: Qualitative test (penta cyano
          ammonioferrate reagent) 1) 21 genera-negative (absences
          of canavanine); 2) 9 genera-positive; 3) Different species
          of *Vicia,* (3 neg., 1 positive); 4) Canavanine in *Medicago
          sativa* metabolized during germination of seed.

50. Bemis, W. P., J. W. Berry, M. J. Kennedy, D. Woods, M.
    Moran and A. J. Deutschman, Jr.

   1967   Oil composition of *Cucurbita.* *J. Amer. Oil Chem. Soc.*
          44:429-430.

          Nutr. Abstr., 38:310.

17

Bemis, W. P., J. W. Berry, M. J. Kennedy, D. Woods, M. Moran and A. J. Deutschman, Jr. (cont.)

Palmitic, stearic, oleic, linoleic and linolenic acid contents in seeds of 17 species of *Curcurbita* including *C. foetidissima. (This species yielded an edible oil)*. Range of 10.9-39.4 percent oil among the various species.

51. Bennett, Emmett

1966 Partial chemical composition of four species of coniferous seeds. *For. Sci.* 12(3):317-318.

Moisture, ash, tot. N, Sol. N, reducing sugar, sucrose, xylan, lignin, ether extract; oil fraction: acid value, saponification value, density (D_{25}), Refractive Index $([n])_D 40$.

Species: *Abies balsamea* L., *A. concolor* (Gord. and Glend), Lindl., *Pinus strobus* L., *Picea glauca* (Moench) Voss.

52. Bennett, Emmet and W. D. Weeks

1960 Hemicelluloses and winter hardiness in raspberry canes. *J. Agric. Food Chem.* 8(4):321.

Hemicellulose composition of Latham and Milton raspberry canes reported on an ash-, moisture- and lignin-free basis.

53. Bentley, R. K., E. R. H. Jones and V. Thaller

1969 Natural acetylenes. 30. Polyacetylenes from Lactuca (lettuce) species of the Liguliflorae subfamily of the Compositae. *J. Chem. Soc.* (C), 7:1096-1099.

54. Bezeau, L. M. and A. Johnston

 1962   *In vitro* digestibility of range forage plants of the *Festuca scabrella* association. *Canad. J. Plant Sci.* 42(4):692-697.

 In vitro digestibility of cellulose determined for 20 grasses, 6 forbs and 6 miscellaneous browse plants of the *Festuca scabrella* association of South Alberta, Canada. The calculation of the nutritive value index (N.V.I.), and the percent digestible protein at 5 stages of growth are also reported.

55. Bezeau, L. M., A. Johnston and S. Smoliak

 1966   Silica and protein content of mixed prairie and fescue grassland vegetation and its relationship to the incidence of silica urolithiasis. *Canad. J. Plant Sci.* 46(6):625-631.

 Percent sand, percent protein, percent silica at 5 stages of growth for 43 species of grasses, sedges, forbs and shrubs in both fescue grassland forage and mixed prairie forage.

56. Biely, J. and W. D. Kitts

 1964   The anti-estrogenic activity of certain legumes and grasses. *Canad. J. Plant Sci.* 44:297-302.

 Nutr. Abstr., 35:3680.

 The anti-estrogen activity of 13 species of legumes and grasses was tested on rats.

57. Billingsley, B. B., Jr. and Dale H. Arner

 1970   The nutritive value and digestibility of some winter foods of the eastern wild turkey. *J. Wildl. Mgmt.* 34(1):176-182.

 Proximate analyses and digestibility.

Billingsley, B. B., Jr. and Dale H. Arner (cont.)

Species: *Cornus florida*, *Vitis aestivalis* (summer grape), *Quercus nigra*, *Smilax rotundifolia*, *Cyperus esculentus*, *Carya illinoensis*, *Celtis laevigata*, *Lindera benzoin*.

58. Binder, R. G., T. H. Applewhite, M. J. Diamond and L. A. Goldblatt

1964 Chromatographic analysis of seed oils. II. Fatty acid composition of *Dimorphotheca* oil. *J. Am. Oil Chemists' Soc.* 41:108-111.

59. Birdsong, B. A., R. Alston and B. L. Turner

1960 Distribution of canavanine in the family Leguminosae as related to phyletic groupings. *Canad. J. Bot.* 38:500.

Qualitative analysis for canavanine of 219 species of 109 genera. Results reported sixty-eight species of 32 genera possess canavanine in their seeds.

60. Bishop, James S. and G. P. Spinner

1946 Quantities of weed seed produced in Connecticut cornfields. *J. Wildl. Mgmt.* 10(4):300-303.

Species: *Ambrosia artemisiifolia*, *Chenopodium album*, *Polygonum pennsylvanicum*, *Echinocloa crus-galli*, *Amaranthus retroflexus*, *Setaria glauca*, *Panicum capillare*, *Digitaria sanguinalis*.

61. Bissell, H. D.

1959 Interpreting chemical analyses of browse. *Calif. Fish and Game* 45(1):57-58.

62. Bissell, H. D. and H. Strong

    1955 The crude protein variations in the browse diet of Cali-
          fornia deer. *Calif. Fish and Game* 41(2):145-155.

63. Blaim, K.

    1962 (Betaine and choline in seeds.) *Rocz. Nauk rol.* (A), 86:
          527-531. Polish: Russian and English summaries.

          Nutr. Abstr., 33:2248.

          Some American species included: eg. *Cucurbita pepo,
          Nicotiana rustica, N. tabacum.*

64. Blair, Robert M. and E. A. Epps, Jr.

    1967 Distribution of protein and phosphorous in spring growth
          of rusty blackhaw. *J. Wildl. Mgmt.* 31(1):188-190.

          Nutr. Abstr., 38:304.

          P and crude protein in various parts of twigs and leaves
          reported.

          Species: *Viburnum rufidulum* (Southern range shrub).

65. Blaisdell, James P., A. C. Wiese and C. W. Hodgson

    1952 Variations in chemical composition of bluebunch wheat-
          grass, arrowleaf balsamroot, and associated range plants.
          J. Range Mgmt. 5(5):346-353.

          For the first two species, results of proximate analyses at
          various times (April-November) over a 4 year period re-
          ported. For the rest, results of proximate analyses give
          variation over 1 year of content of crude protein, Ca, P
          and Ca/P ratio.

21

Blaisdell, James P., A. C. Wiese and C. W. Hodgson (cont.)

Species: *Agropyron spicatum, Balsamorhiza sagittata, Crepis acuminata, Purshia tridentata, Poa secunda, Artemisia tripartita.*

66. Block, R. J. and K. W. Weiss

1956 Amino acid handbook, 1st ed., Charles C. Thomas, Springfield, Illinois.

67. Boag, D. A. and J. W. Kiceniuk

1968 Protein and caloric content of lodgepole pine needles. *Forestry Chronicle* 44(4):28-31.

68. Boggino, Eloy, J. A.

1970 Chemical composition and in vitro dry master digestibility of range grasses. Unpublished M.S. thesis, New Mexico State University, Las Cruces, 134 pages

69. Bohmont, Bert L. and Robert Lang

1957 Some variations in morphological characteristics and palatability among geographic strains of Indian ricegrass. *J. Range Mgmt.* 10(3):127-131.

Species: *Oryzopsis hymenoides.*

70. Bohn, H. L. and M. M. Aba-Husayn

1971 Manganese, iron, copper and zinc concentrations of *Sporobolus wrightii* in alkaline soils. *Soil Sci.* 112(5): 348-350.

In situ sampling of alkali sacaton grass: 1) pH 7.5-9.5:

Bohn, H. L. and M. M. Aba-Husayn (cont.)

levels of Cu and Zn decreased with increasing soil pH and levels of Fe and Mn increased with increasing soil pH. 2) Linear regression equins relating ion concentrations in plants to soil pH: Mn -40.1 + 6.41 pH (R^2 = 0.348); Fe = -258 + 47.7 pH (R^2 = 0.592); Cu = 19.0 - 1.66 pH (R^2 = 0.348); Zn = 50.7 - 4.77 pH (R^2 = 0.719).

71. Bollard, E. G.

1957 Composition of the nitrogen fraction of apple tracheal sap. *Austral. J. Biol. Sci.* 10:279-287.

1) Amounts of various nitrogenous compounds and total N in tracheal sap from apple treas (ug N/ml sap). 2) Proportions of various nitrogenous compounds present in apple tracheal sap for Granny Smith trees during the growing season (various amino acids).

72. −.

1957 Nitrogenous compounds in tracheal sap of woody members of the family *Rosaceae. Austral. J. Biol. Sci.* 10: 288-291.

Amounts of various nitrogenous compounds in tracheal sap from trees (ammonia N, glutamineamide N, aspargine aneride N, amino N, tot. ammonia amide and amino nitrogen and tot. Kjeldahl N), also tabulated are amino acid quantities. All species sampled in September-December, 1954.

Species: Pear, quince, Japanese plum, Myrobalan plum, peach, apricot, flowering cherry and apple.

73. −.

1957 Translocation of organic nitrogen in the xylem. *Austral.*

Bollard, E. G. (cont.)

J. Biol. Sci. 10:292-301.

1) Xylem sap Nitrogen content and that of 15 other compounds present in xylem sap determined for 31 genera of dicots, 6 genera of monocots and 9 genera of gymnosperms. 2) Semiquantitative determination of citrulline, allantoin, and allantoic acid in the xylem sap of 30 genera reported.

74. Bondi, A. and H. Meyer

1948   Lignins in young plants. *Biochem. J.* 43:248.

Analysis of lignins in 4 grasses and 4 legumes.

75. Borell, A. E.

1951   Russian olive as a wildlife food. *J. Wildl. Mgmt.* 15(1): 109-110.

Proximate analysis, Ca and P of fruit.

Species: *Eleagnus angustifolia L.*

76. Bovey, R. W., D. Le Tourneau and L. C. Erickson

1961   The chemical composition of medusahead and downy brome. *Weeds* 9(2):307-311.

77. Bowden, D. M., D. K. Taylor and W. E. P. Davis

1968   Water-soluble carbohydrates in orchard-grass and mixed forages. *Canad. J. Plant Sci.* 48:9-15.

78. Bowman, D. E. and A. G. Law

    1964 Effects of temperature and daylength on the development
          of lignin, cellulose, and protein in *Dactylis glomerata* L.
          and *Bromis inermis* Leyss. *Agron. J.* 56:177-179.

          Nutr. Abstr., 35:328.

79. Boyd, C. E.

    1968 Evaluation of some common aquatic weeds as possible
          feedstuffs. *Hyacinth Control J.* 7:26-27.

80. —.

    1969 The nutritive value of three species of water weeds. *Econ.
          Bot.* 23:123-127.

          P, S, Ca, Mg, K, dry matter, crude protein, cellulose, tot.
          available CHO, ether extract, ash, caloric content, and
          amino acid content.

          Species: *Eichhornia crassipes, Pistia stratiotes* and
          Hydrilla sp.

81. —.

    1970 Amino acid, protein, and caloric content of vascular
          aquatic macrophytes. *Ecology* 51:902-906.

          Lush green vegetative material harvested during April-
          July: Comparison of amino acid analyses of *Typha
          latifolia* (g/100g protein) and protein and caloric con-
          tent of 11 aquatic species reported.

          *Typha latifolia, Hydrotrida carolinensis, Brasenia schre-
          beri, Utricularia inflata, Nelumbo lutea, Myriophyllum
          heterophyllum, Eleocharis acicularis, Najas guadalupensis,
          Nymphaea odorata, Ceratophyllum demersum, Nuphar
          adrena.*

25

82. —.

1970 Chemical analysis of some vascular aquatic plants. *Archiv. Hydrobiol.* 67:78-85.

83. —.

1970 Losses of mineral nutrients during decomposition of *Typha latifolia. Archiv. Hydrobiol.* 66:511-517.

84. —.

1970 Production, mineral accumulation and pigment concentration in *Typha latifolia* and *Scirpus americanus. Ecology* 51(2):285-290.

1) Moisture content over time, carotenoids, chlorophyll A and chlor. B (mg/gm pigments (dry wt.); 2) Shoot productivity/April-July percent composition of ash, N, P, S, Ca, Mg, K and Na and gms/m^2 in *Typha* stands and *Scirpus* stands; 3) Carbon content of dry matter (%) over a period of time; and dry matter production over time (g/m^2); 4) Rates of uptake (mg/m^2/day) of nutrients; 5) N, P, S, Ca, Mg, K, and Na (%) given for *Typha* fruits.

85. —.

1970 Vascular aquatic plants for mineral nutrient removal from polluted waters. *Econ. Bot.* 24(1):95-103.

Mean mineral nutrient composition of dried samples of water plants from young stands include ash percent, N percent, P (%), S (%), Ca (%), Mg (%), K (%), Na (%), Fe (ppm), Mn (ppm), Zn (ppm), Cu (ppm).

Species: *Eichhornia crassipes, Justicia americana, Alternanthera philoxeroides, Typha latifolia.*

86. Boyd, C. E. and J. M. Lawrence

   1966   The mineral composition of several freshwater algae. *Proc. Ann. Conf., S. E. Assn., Game and Fish Comm.* 20:413-424.

87. Boyd, C. E. and L. W. Hess

   1970   Factors influencing shoot production and mineral nutrient levels in Typha latifolia. *Ecology* 51:295-300.

   1) Positive correlation of standing crop with dilute acid-soluble P in hydrosoils and dissolved P in waters; 2) Weak correlation for dissolved Ca and shoot production; 3) Frequency distributions given for concentrations (%) of ash, carbon, N, P, Ca, Mg, K, Na and S in tissues; and 4) Correlation between N and Ash, P, S. and K.

88. Boyd, C. E. and R. D. Blackburn

   1970/71   Seasonal changes in the proximate composition of some common aquatic weeds. *Hyacinth Control J.*

89. Boyd, Claude E.

   1968   Fresh-water plants: A potential source of protein. *Econ. Bot.* 22:359-368.

   Leaf protein extraction data and protein yields for 20 aquatic species; mean nutritional analyses of leaf protein (ash, crude fat, cellulose and caloric content), essential amino acid composition of aquatic plant leaf protein, amount of pulp dry matter retained as fiber after extraction and nutritional analysis of fiber.

   Species: *Justicia americana, Orontium, aquaticum, Nymphaea odorata, Sagittaria latifolia and Alternanthera philoxeroides;* also: dry matter and proximate analyses (plus cellulose and tannin) for 12 species of submersed vascular plants, 20 species of emergent vascular plants, 8 species of algae and the crude protein contents of 14 species of vascular aquatic plants are reported.

90. Bradfield, R. B. and A. Roca

   1964   Camu-camu—a fruit high in ascorbic acid. *J. Amer. Die-*

27

Bradfield, R. B. and A. Roca (cont.)

tetic Assn. 44:28-30.

Nutr. Abstr., 34:4026.

Myrciaria paraensis Berg found along rivers of the Amazon basin.

91. Bradshaw, A. D., R. W. Lodge, D. Jowett and M. J. Chadwick

1958 Experimental investigations into the mineral nutrition of several grass species. Part 1. Calcium level. *J. Ecol.* 46: 749-757.

Six species of grasses grown in different concentrations of Ca periodically harvested and analyzed. Results reported for root and shoot Ca levels (reported in shoot:root ratio).

92. Branes, L. and E. Ballester

1969 Studies on some toxic substances in *Brassica napus* L. var. Winter Rape, cultivated in Chile. *Qual. Plant. Materiae Vegetabiles* 17:257-264.

Nutr. Abstr., 40:4767.

93. Bravo, F. O.

1971 (Chemical composition of the seeds of *Clitoria ternata* L.). *Tecnica Pecuariaen Mexico* 18:100-102. Spanish: English Summary.

Nutr. Abstr., 42:5327

Proximate contents Ca levels, P levels and some tannin and amino acid components reported.

94. Bressani, R. and R. Arroyave

   1963 Essential amino acid content and protein value of pump-
        kin seed *(Cucurbita farinosa). J. Agric. Food Chem.* 11:
        29-33.

        Nutr. Abstr., 33:4175.

        Proximate composition and essential amino acid content
        tabulated.

95. Brown, E. M.

   1943 Seasonal variations in the growth and chemical composi-
        tion of certain pasture grasses. Missouri Agr. Exp. Sta.
        Res. *Bulletin,* 299, 56 pages.

96. Buck, C. C.

   1938 Progress report on variations in the moisture content of
        green brush foliage on the Shasta Experimental Forest
        during 1937. Calif. For. and Range Expt. Sta., unpub-
        lished manuscript.

97. —.

   1939 Progress report on variations in the moisture content of
        green brush foliage on the Shasta Experimental Forest
        during 1938. Calif. For and Range Expt. Sta., unpub-
        lished manuscript.

98. Bujard, E. and J. Mauron

   1963 (Nutrition problems posed by the struggle against protein
        malnutrition in developing countries. 4. Content of
        amino acids of Para nuts, *Bertholletia excelsa* (Humb. et.
        Bonpl.). An interesting source of methionine for north-
        east Brazil). *Ann. Nutr. Alimentation* 17:73-80. In

Bujard, E. and J. Mauron (cont.)

French.

Nutr. Abstr., 34:277.

99. Burkitt, William H.

1940 The apparent digestibility and nutritive value of beardless wheatgrass at three stages of maturity. *J. Agric. Res.* 61(6):471-479.

Proximate content, Ca, P, and digestibility.

Species: *Agropyron inerme* (Scribn. and Smith) Rydb.

100. Burns, J. C., C. H. Noller and C. L. Rhykerd

1964 Influence of method of drying on the soluble carbohydrate content of alfalfa. *Agron. J.* 56:364-365.

Evidence suggesting significant differences between oven-dried and freeze-dried samples with respect to the soluble carbohydrate content derived from subsequent biochemical analyses.

101. Burns, J. C. and W. F. Wedin

1964 Yield and chemical composition of sudangrass and forage sorghum under three systems of summer management for late fall *in situ* utilization. *Agron. J.* 56:457-460.

102. Burns, R. E.

1963 Plant sources of cellulase for testing cellulase inhibitors in forages. *Agron. J.* 55:374-375.

Nutr. Abstr., 34:2177.

Burns, R. E. (cont.)

    Species: Alfalfa and *Cynodon*.

103. —.

    1966   Tannin in *Sericea lespedeza*. Georgia Agric. Exp. Sta. *Bulletin*, No. N.S. 164, p. 17, June.

    Nutr. Abstr., 38:2384.

104. Burton, G. W.

    1954   Does disease resistance affect forage quality? *Agron. J.* 46:99.

    Proximate contents, lignin, cellulose, Ca and P in disease-free and *Collectotricum graminicola* (antracnose) infected plants of sudangrass.

    Species: Sudangrass.

105. Burzlaff, D. F.

    1971   Seasonal variations of the in vitro dry-matter digestibility of three sandhill grasses. *J. Range Mgmt.* 24(1):60-63.

    Both digestibility and crude protein content declined in all grasses with advance in maturity.

    Species: *Andropogon hallii* Hack, *A. scoparius* Mich, *Calamovilfa longifolia* (Hook.) Scribn.

106. Butler, G. W., P. C. Barclay and A. C. Glenday

    1962   Genetic and environmental differences in the mineral composition of rye grass herbage. *Plant and Soil* 16:214-228.

Butler, G. W., P. C. Barclay and A. C. Glenday (cont.)

Differences in mineral content and growth of herbage from 7 ryegrass clones. ppm: Zn, Fe, Ti, Cu, Al, Mn; mg %: Ca, K, Na, Sulphate-S, Acid Soluble P, Nitrate-N. Also genetic correlations for differences in mineral composition, growth and root cation-exchange capacity reported. Authors found significant heritabilities for all nutrients except K.

107. Butterworth, M. H.

1968 Una nota sobre el contenido de proteina cruda en pasto pangola (*Digitaria decumbens stent*) bajo diferentes sistemas de manejo. (Crude protein content of pangola grass (*Digitaria decumbens stent*) under different systems of management). *Rev. Mex. Prod. Animal* 1:29-31. Spanish: English Summary.

Nutr. Abstr., 40:2553.

108. Buttery, R. F. and J. H. Ehrenreich

1961 Nutritive quality of little bluestem in the Missouri Ozarks. Central States For. Exp. Sta. *Tech. Paper*, 179, 9 pp.

109. Byers, M.

1971 Amino acid composition and *in vitro* digestibility of some protein fractions from three species of leaves of various ages. *J. Sci. Food Agric.* 22(5):242-251.

Nutr. Abstr., 42:314.

Species: Barley, lupin, chinese cabbage.

110. Byrd, Morris, W. C. Young and V. E. Davison

1963   Seed yields of shrub Lespedezas in Arkansas. *J. Wildl. Mgmt.* 27(1):135-136.

lbs/acre yields for *Lespedeza japonica* and *L. bicolor* grown on experimental plots.

C

111. Cable, Dwight R. and J. W. Bohning

1959   Changes in grazing use and herbage content of three exotic lovegrasses and some native grasses. *J. Range Mgmt.* 12(4):200-203.

Species: *Eragrostis lehmanniana, E. chloromelas, E. superba;* also *Trichachne californica, Bouteloua hirsuta, B. curtipendula, Heteropogon contortus.*

112. Cable, Dwight T. and R. P. Shumway

1966   Crude protein in rumen contents and in forage. *J. Range Mgmt.* 19(3):124-128.

Trichachne californica (Benth.) Chase, *Eragrostis lehmanniana* Nees; *Zinnia pumila* Gray; *Opuntia fulgida* Engel.; *O. engelmannii* Salm-Dyck; *Prosopis juliflora* var. *velutina* (Woot.) Sarg. crude protein % in dry matter; monthly averages May, 1961-September, 1963.

113. Cain, J. C.

1959   I. Factors in sampling and analysis for the diagnosis of nutritional status of trees. II. Observations on antagonis-

Cain, J. C. (cont.)

tic effects in leaf analysis. Duke Univ. School of Forestry *Bulletin*, 15:55-70.

114. Cain, John C.

1959   Plant tissues analysis: Part II. Observations on antagonistic effects in leaf analysis. Duke Univ. School Forestry *Bulletin*, 15:63-70.

A discussion of relationships between N, K, Mg and P. Results of experimentation indicate that with Nitrogen fertilization the K and P content of leaves decreases while the Mg content increases. With K fertilization the Mg content of the leaves decreases. Author discusses a possible mechanism.

115. Cairnie, A. G. and J. C. Monesiglio

1967   (Chemical composition of native and introduced forage species in the semi-arid region of La Pampa.). *Rev. Invest. Agropecuar.* Ser. 2,4¾207-221. Spanish: English Summary.

Nutr. Abstr., 38:2326.

The chemical composition of 32 native and introduced forage species and 7 cereal grains is reported.

116. Campbell, R. S., E. A. Epps, Jr., C. C. Moreland, J. L. Farr and F. Bonner

1954   Nutritive values of native plants on forest range in Central Louisiana. La. Agr. Exp. Sta. *Bulletin*, 488, 18 pp.

117. Cannon, T. F., L. C. Chadwick and K. W. Reisch

1960 The nutrient element status of some ornamental trees. *Proc. Amer. Soc Hort. Sci.* 76:661-666.

Report on the N, P, K, Ca, Mg, Fe and Mn content of mid-shoot leaves for the months of June, July, August, and September of *Crataegus phaenopyrum, Quercus palustris,* and *Gleditsia triacanthos inermis.*

118. Carter, D. L., M. J. Brown, W. H. Allaway and E. E. Cary

1968 Selenium content of forage and hay crops in the Pacific Northwest. *Agronomy J.* 60:532-534.

Nutr. Abstr., 39:6717.

119. Carter, M. C. and E. S. Lyle, Jr.

1966 Fertilization of loblolly pine on two Alabama soils: Effect on growth and foliar mineral content. Ala. Agr. Exp. Sta. *Bulletin,* 370, Auburn.

120. Carter, Mason C. and H. S. Larsen

1965 Soil nutrients and loblolly pine xylem sap composition. *For. Sci.* 11(2):217-220.

Experimental stands treated with fertilizers of N, P, and K in the following combinations: N, P, NP, K, NK, PK and NPK. The xylem sap of the treated trees was then analyzed for micromoles per ml, Total-N, Amide-N, Amino-N (ppm), P (ppm), and K (ppm).

121. Castillo, Y.

1965 (Lupins ["Chocho"] in Ecuador.) *Arch. Venz. Nutricion* 15:87-93. Spanish: English Summary.

Castillo, Y. (cont.)

Nutr. Abstr., 37:299.

Proximate comp. and Ca, P, Fe, carotene, vit. B, ritbofla-
vin, nicotinic acid.

Species: *Lupinus tricolor* and *L. mutabilis* both are high
alt. species of the Andes. Preparation: boiled 12 hours,
washed 7-8 days. The bitter principle is an alkaloid.

122. Catlin, C. N.

1925 Composition of Arizona forages with comparative data.
Arizona Agr. Exp. Sta. *Bulletin,* 113.

123. Chatfield, C. and G. Adams

1940 Proximate composition of American food materials.
U.S.D.A. circular 549.

Only part of this publication has been included in Watt
and Merrill USDA Handbook 8; a number of wild foods
included in circular 549 were deleted from the Handbook
8 and for this reason it is listed here as a separate reference.

124. Chatterton, N. J., J. R. Goodin, C. M. McKell, R. V. Parker and J. M. Rible

1971 Monthly variation in the chemical composition of desert
saltbush. *J. Range Mgmt.* 24(1):37-40.

Nutr. Abstr., 42:2967.

Analysis (Proximate); Ca and P content of leaves and new
and old stems of edible size.

Species: *Atriplex polycarpa* (Torr.) S. Wats.

36

125. Chenault, Tandy P.

1940 The phenology of some Bob-White food and cover plants in Brazos County, Texas. *J. Wildl. Mgmt.* 4(4):359-368.

Tabulation of developmental cycle (with dates) for approximately 90 types of plants.

126. Chenery, E. M.

1955 A preliminary study of aluminum and the tea bush. *Plant and Soil* 6:174-200.

Diverse geographic varieties are analyzed for the Al, Mn, and P content of various vegetative portions. The effects of pH, leaf age, genetics, and interaction of Mn and P with Al on exchangeable Al are considered.

Species: *Camellia sinensis.*

127. Childers, N. F.

1954 *Fruit Nutrition.* Somerset Press, Somerville, N.J., 907 pp.

The subject: mineral nutrition of specific fruit crops.

128. Chisholm, M. J. and C. Y. Hopkins

1964 Fatty acid composition of some Cucurbitaceae seed oils. *Canad. J. Chem.* 42:560-564.

Nutr. Abstr., 34:5587.

129. Christensen, F. W. and T. H. Hopper

1932 Effect of weathering and stage of maturity on the palatibility and nutritive value of prairie hay. N. Dak. Agr. Exp. Sta. *Bulletin,* 260, 55 pp.

130. Christenson, F. W., T. H. Hopper and O. A. Stevens

1948 Digestible nutrients and metabolizable energy in Russian-thistle hays and silages. *J. Agr. Res.* 76:73-93.

Proximate contents and P of samples taken on various soils and at various stages of maturity. Differences among leaves, stems and floral tips for one collection reported along with proximate contents of various mixed silages and results of using these in metabolism trials on sheep.

Species: *Salsola kali* L.

131. Christisen, D. M.

1951 Yield of acorns from a post oak, *Quercus stellata*, August, 1949, Indian Trail Refuge, Dent County, Missouri. *J. Wildl. Mgmt.* 15(3):332-333.

132. —.

1955 Yield of seed by oaks in the Missouri Ozarks. *J. Forestry* 53(6):439-441.

133. Christisen, D. M. and L. J. Korschgen

1955 Acorn yields and wildlife usage in Missouri. *Trans. N. Amer. Wildl. Conf.* 20:337-356.

134. Clarke, S. E. and E. W. Tisdale

1945 The chemical composition of native forage plants of Southern Alberta and Saskatchewan in relation to grazing practices. Canad. Dept. Agr. *Tech. Bulletin,* 54.

135. Collins, J. O.

1961   Ten year acorn mast production study in Louisiana. Louisiana Wild Life and Fisheries Comm. P. R. *Rept.* Project W-29-R-8, 33 pp.

136. Cook, C. W.

1966   Carbohydrate reserve in plants.   Utah Agr. Exp. Sta. Utah *Resources Series* 31, 47 pp.

137. Cook, C. W., L. A. Stoddart and L. E. Harris

1952   Determining the digestibility and metabolizable energy of winter range plants by sheep. *J. Anim. Sci.* 11:578-590.

Dry wt. proximate contents (crude fiber divided into percent lignin, percent cellulose); also percent Ca and P reported. The digestibility (by sheep) of each species is compared against timothy hay and alfalfa on the basis of gross energy, energy loss, and metabolizable energy (these calculated on a dry wt. basis).

Species: *Artemisia nova,* (black sage); *Atriplex confertifolia* (shadscale); *Artemsia tridentata,* (big sagebrush); *Sitanion hystrix,* (Squirrel tail grass).

138. Cook, C. W., L. A. Stoddart and L. E. Harris

1954   The nutritive value of winter range plants in the Great Basin.   Utah State Agr. Coll. Exp. Sta. *Bulletin,* 372, 56 pp.

139. —.

1959   The chemical content in various portions of the current growth of salt-desert shrubs and grasses during winter.

Cook, C. W., L. A. Stoddart and L. E. Harris (cont.)

Ecology 40:644-651.

Four intensities of harvest analyzed for proximate contents, lignin, cellulose, Ca and P.

Species: *Artemisia nova, Eurotia lanata, Kochia vestita, Ephedra nevadensis, Atriplex canescens, Chrysothamnus stenophyllus, Sporobolus cryptandrus, Atriplex confertifolia, Stipa comata, Hilaria jamesii, Oryzopsis hymenoides.*

140. Cook, C. W. and L. E. Harris

1950   The nutritive content of the grazing sheep's diet on summer and winter ranges of Utah. Utah Agr. Exp. Sta. *Bulletin,* 342, 66 pp.

141. —.

1950   The nutritive value of range forage as affected by vegetation type, site and stage of maturity. Utah Agr. Exp. Sta. Tech. *Bulletin,* 344, 45 pp.

142. Cook, C. Wayne

1959   The effect of site on the palatability and nutritive content of seeded wheatgrasses. *J. Range Mgmt.* 12(6):289-292.

For three species of *Agropyron,* proximate analyses of plants growing on favorable and unfavorable sites are reported. Leaves, stems and whole plants are treated separately.

143. Cook, C. Wayne, L. A. Stoddart and L. E. Harris

1951   Measuring consumption and digestibility of winter range

Cook, C. Wayne, L. A. Stoddart and L. E. Harris (cont.)

plants by sheep. *J. Range Mgmt.* 4(5):335-346.

Proximate content.

Species: *Atriplex nuttallii, A. confertifolia, Eurotia lanata, Artemisia tridentata, A. nova, Sitanion hystrix,* alfalfa.

144. —.

1953 Effects of grazing intensity upon the nutritive value of range forage. *J. Anim. Science.*

Proximate analyses.

Species: *Atriplex confertifolia, Artemisia nova.*

145. Cook, C. Wayne and L. E. Harris

1952 Nutritive value of cheatgrass and crested wheatgrass on spring ranges of Utah. *J. Range Mgmt.* 5(5):331-337.

Proximate analyses.

Species: *Bromus tectorum* and *Agropyron* sp.

146. Coyne, P. I.

1969 Seasonal trend in total available carbohydrates with respect to phenological stage of development in eight desert range species. Unpublished Ph.D. dissert., Utah State Univ., Logan, Utah, 164 pp.

147. Coyne, Patrick I and C. W. Cook

1970 Seasonal carbohydrate reserve cycles in eight desert range

Coyne, Patrick I. and C. W. Cook (cont.)

species. *J. Range Mgmt.* 23(6):438-444.

Species: *Artemisia tridentata, A. arbuscula* var. *nova., Atriplex confertifolia, A. falcata, Eurotia lanata, Oryzopsis hymenoides, Stipa comata, Sitanion hystrix.*

148. Crampton, E. W. and R. Forshaw

1940   Pasture studies XVI. The nutritive values of Kentucky blue grass, red top and brome grass. *J. Nutrition* 19(2): 161-172.

Proximate content, lignin, cellulose and other carbohydrate components reported for various stages of maturity.

149. Crooke, W. M. and A. H. Knight

1962   An evaluation of published data on the mineral composition of plants in the light of the cation-exchange capacities of their roots. *Soil Sci.* 93:365-373.

Changes in the proximate contents of the tops of plants with an increase in ash content are reported. Major- and trace-element contents of various pasture plants and weeds are reported as well.

150. Crooke, W. M., A. H. Knight and J. Keay

1964   Mineral composition, cation-exchange properties and uronic acid content of various tissues of conifers. *For. Sci.* 10(4):415-427.

Analyses of needles, stems, roots, seeds and pollen. 1) Cation-exchange capacity, excess base, uronic acid content, ash, N and Fe (for tissue of seedlings); 2) Ash, K, Ca, Uronic acid, cation-exchange capacity, Mg, N, P, S, Cl, total anions, and excess base (for pine needles);

Crooke, W. M., A. H. Knight and J. Keay (cont.)

3) Mineral analyses of pollen.

Species: *Abies* (4 spp.), *Cedrus* (2 spp.), *Chamaecyparis* (1 sp.), *Cupressus* (1 sp.), *Juniperus* (1 sp.); *Larix* (2 spp.); *Picea* (3 spp.); *Pinus* (5 spp.); *Pseudotsuga* (1 sp.); *Metasequoia* (1 sp.); *Sequoia* (2 spp.); *Taxus* (1 sp.); *Thuja* (1 sp.) and *Tsuga* (1 sp.).

151. Cypert, E. and B. S. Webster

1948   Yield and use by wild life of acorns of water and willow oaks. *J. Wildl. Mgmt.* 12(3):227-231.

Report on quantities of mast produced in relation to tree age and size.

Species: *Quercus nigra*, (water oak); *Q. phellos*, (willow oak).

D

152. Dalke, P. D.

1953   Yields of seeds and mast in second growth hardwood forest, South-central Missouri. *J. Wildl. Mgmt.* 17(3): 378-380.

Summary of seed and mast yield on 452 mil -acre plots in the fall of 1938 and 494 mil -acre plots in the fall of 1939.

Species: *Quercus velutina, Q. alba, Q. coccinea, Q. rubra, Q. borealis, Rosa* sp., *Q. stellata, Q. marilandica, Lespedeza virginica, Symphoricarpos orbiculatus, Carya*

Dalke, P. D. (cont.)

sp., *Rhus* sp., *Corylus americana, Cornus florida, Ceanothus americanus.*

153. Dalke, Paul D. and P. R. Sime

1941   Food habits of the eastern and New England cottontails. *J. Wildl. Mgmt.* 5(2):216-228.

Proximate analyses reported of the barks of 24 woody plants consumed by cottontail rabbits.

154. Dalrymple, R. L., D. D. Dwyer and J. E. Webster

1965   Cattle utilization and chemical content of winged elm browse. *J. Range Mgmt.* 18(3):126-128.

Proximate analysis of twigs reported along with analyses of lignin, sugars, acid hydrolysis, alcohol-soluble solids, nitrogen and ash.

Species: *Ulmus alata.*

155. Daniel, H. A. and H. J. Harper

1934   The relation between total calcium and phosphorous in mature prairie grass and available plant food in the soil. *J. Amer. Soc. Agron.* 26(12):986-992.

156. Daniel, Harley A.

1934   The calcium phosphorous and nitrogen content of grasses and legumes; and the relation of these elements in the plant. *Agron. J.* 26:496-503.

Percent Ca, N and P, and the ratios Ca:P, N:Ca and N:P for 25 grasses and 12 legumes.

157. Davidson, H.

1960 Nutrient element composition of leaves from selected species of ornamental plants. *Proc. Ameri. Soc. Hort. Sci.* 76:667-671.

Elements reported: N, P, K, Ca, Mg, B, Fe, Cu, Mn (for the months of June, July, and August).

Species: *Gleditsia triacanthos, Acer platanoides, Syringa vulgaris, Euonymus alatus, Juniperus chinensis, Euonymus fortunei.*

158. Daxenbichler, M. E., C. H. Van Etten, H. Zobel and I. A. Wolff

1962 Isothiocyanates from enzymatic hydrolysis of *Lesquerella* seed meals. *J. Am. Oil Chemists' Soc.* 39(5):244-245.

159. Daxenbichler, M. E., C. H. Van Etten and I. A. Wolff

1965 A new thioglucoside, (*R*)-2-hydroxy-3-butenylglucosinolate from *Crambe abyssinica* seed. *Biochem.* 4(2):318-323.

160. —.

1968 Diastereomeric episulfides from *Epi*-progoitrin upon autolysis of crambe seed meal. *Phytochemistry* 7(6):989-996.

161. Daxenbichler, M. E., C. H. Van Etten, W. H. Tallent and I. A. Wolff

1967 Rapeseed meal autolysis. Formation of diastereomeric (2*R*)-1-Cyano-2-hydroxy-3, 4 epithiobutanes from progoitrin. *Canad. J. Chem.* 45(17):1971-1974.

162. Daxenbichler, Melvin E., C. H. Van Etten, E. A. Hallinan, F. R. Earle and A. S. Barclay

> 1971   Seeds as sources of L-Dopa. *J. Med. Chem.* 14(5):463-465.
>
> A discussion of various genera of the Leguminosae.

163. Daxenbichler, Melvin E., C. H. Van Etten and I. A. Wolff

> 1961   Identification of a new, naturally occurring, steam-volatile isothiocyanate from *Lesquerella lasiocarpa* seed. *J. Org. Chem.* 26(10):4168-4169.

164. de Bruin, A.

> 1964   Investigation of the food value of quinua and canihua seed. *J. Food Sci.* 29:872-876.
>
> Nutr. Abstr., 35:3631.
>
> Proximate contents, saponin, analyses of carbohydrates, analyses of N compounds, 16 minerals, vit. B_1, nicotinic acid, tocopherol, ascorbic acid, carotenoids, P:Ca ratio.
>
> Species: *Chenopodium quinoa* and *C. pallidicaule* grown in Holland.

165. Dee, Richard F. and T. W. Box

> 1967   Commercial fertilizers influence crude protein content of four mixed prairie grasses. *J. Range Mgmt.* 20(1):96-99.
>
> Percent crude protein reported under various treatments of N-fertilizer for the months of September through March.
>
> Species: *Chloris verticellata* Nutt., *Bouteloua gracilis*

Dee, Richard F. and T. W. Box (cont.)

HBK., *Buchloe dactyloides* Nutt., and *Andropogon saccharoides* Swartz.

166. Demarchi, Raymond A.

1968　Chemical composition of bighorn winter forages. *J Range Mgmt.* 21(6):385-388.

Proximate analyses, Ca and P.

Species: *Agropyron spicatum, Stipa columbiana, Koeleria cristata, Poa secunda, Eriogonum heracleoides, Achillea millefolium, Artemisia frigida,* Idaho fescue.

167. DeRiveros, M. H. C. K. and E. E. Vonesch

1969　Determinacion *in vitro* de algunos nutrientes en cinco forrajeras cultivadas en la Republica Argentina. (Estimation *in vitro* of some nutrients in 5 forages cultivated in the Argentine Republic.) *Rev. Fac. Agronom. Vet.,* Buenos Aires, 17(2):19-24.

Nutr. Abstr., 40:6086.

Proximate analyses.

Species: *Phalaris, Agropyron, Lolium, Dactylis,* and *Medicago* species.

168. Devadas, R. P., V. Anuradha and U. Chandrasekhar

1969　Seasonal variation in the nutrient content of *Amaranthus flavus. J. Nutrition Dietetics,* India, 6:305-307.

Nutr. Abstr., 40:4766.

Protein, Ca, P, Fe and Vitamin C content of leaves.

169. DeWitt, J. B. and J. V. Derby, Jr.

1955   Changes in the nutritive values of browse plants following forest fire. *J. Wildl. Mgmt.* 19(1):65-70.

Proximate contents of browse at different stages of maturity.

Species: *Acer rubrum, Quercus alba, Cornus florida, Smilax rotundifolia* collected on both burned and unburned plots.

170. Dexter, S. T., C. W. Duncan and C. F. Huffman

1957   Nutritional value of sunchoke silage for milk production. *Agron. J.* 49:336-338.

Proximate content, digestibility and comparative value for milk production.

Species: Sunchoke silage (the sunchoke is a cross between artichokes and sunflowers), corn silage, artichoke silage and sunflower silage.

171. Diamond, M. J., R. E. Knowles, R. G. Binder and L. A. Goldblatt

1964   Hydroxy unsaturated oils II. Preparation and characterization of methyl dimorphecolate and methyl lesquerolate from *Dimorphotheca* and *Lesquerella* oils. *J. Am. Oil Chemists' Soc.* 41:430-433.

172. Diaz, H. B.

1962   (Common species of trees which serve as feed for livestock in the livestock regions of the province of Tucuman.) *Turrialba* 12:195-199. Spanish: English Summary.

Nutr. Abstr., 33:4173.

48

Diaz, H. B. (cont.)

> Proximate components of leaves and/or fruits of 20 trees eaten in dry season by livestock.

173. Dietz, D. R.

> 1958 Exploratory analysis of browse samples. Colorado Game and Fish Dept., P-R rept., Project W-38-R-11, 37 pp.

174. Dietz, D. R., R. H. Udall, H. R. Shepherd and L. E. Yeager

> 1958 Seasonal progression in chemical content of five key browse species in Colorado. *Proc. Soc. Am. Foresters*, pp. 117-122.
>
> Crude protein, crude fat, crude fiber, P, carotene, Ca, N-free extract, ash, Ca/P ratio (oven dry basis).
>
> Species: *Quercus gambelli, Purshia tridentata, Artemisia tridentata, Amelanchier alnifolia, Cercocarpus montanus.*

175. Dietz, D. R., R. H. Udall and L. E. Yeager

> 1962 Chemical composition and digestibility by mule deer of selected forage species, Cache la Poudre Range, Colorado. Colorado Game and Fish Dept., *Tech. Publ.* 14, 89 pp.

176. Dietz, Donald R. and R. D. Curnow

> 1966 How reliable is a forage chemical analysis? *J. Range Mgmt.* 19(6):374-376.
>
> Protein, phosphorous, ash and calcium—results of 4 labs compared.
>
> Species: *Populus tremuloides* Mich.

177. Dimbleby, G. W.

1952   The root sap of birch on a podzol. *Plant and Soil* 4:141.

Ca, K, Mn, Na, Fe, Mg, ammonia-N, pH (all in ppm/c.c. of sap), given for the roots of *Betula pubescens* sampled during May to July, and a comparison made of concentrations of Ca, Mg, Na, K, Fe, Mn, and NH_3 (ppm) sampled at the same time for deep and shallow roots. For months of May and June, K, P and Ca are compared for roots from brown forest soil and podzol soil. Also an analysis of sap from pine roots (shallow) is reported.

178. Dirschl, Herman J.

1963   Food habits of the pronghorn in Saskatchewan. *J. Wildl. Mgmt.* 27(1):81-93.

Crude protein content (on a monthly basis) of *Artemisia cana, Juniperus horizontalis, Symphoricarpos occidentalis, Rosa* sp., *Tragopogon dubius.* Kjeldahl procedure (6.25 used as conversion factor for N).

179. Dirven, J. G. P.

1963   The nutritive value of the indigenous grasses of Surinam. *Netherlands J. Agric. Sci.* 11:295-307.

Nutr. Abstr., 34:2158.

Proximate content, K, S, Mg, Cl, Ca, P and Cu.

180. Dirven, J. G. P. and V. K. R. Ehrencron

1963   (Dry matter contents of grasses in the human tropics.) *Surinaamse Landbouw* 11:88-93. Dutch: English Summary.

Nutr. Abstr., 34:2160.

Dirven, J. G. P. and V. K. R. Ehrencron (cont.)

Species: *Paspalum repens, Pennisetum purpureum, Tripsacum laxum, Saccharum sinense* var. *Uba., Cynodon dactylon,* Pangola grass, etc.

181. Dodd, Jimmie D. and H. H. Hopkins

1958   Yield and carbohydrate content of blue grama grass as affected by clipping. *Tran. Kansas Acad. Sci.* 61:280-287.

182. Dominguez, Xorge Alejundro, P. Rojas, V. Collins and M. Del Refugio Morales

1960   A phytochemical study of eight Mexican plants. *Econ. Bot.* 14:157-159.

Leaves, stems, fruits analyzed for alkaloids, saponins, flavones and tannins.

Species: *Xanthium orientale, Amaranthus retroflexus, Notholaena sinuata* var. *cochisensis, Melia azerderach, Cordia boissieri, Jatropha spatulata, Agave schottii, Asclepias erosa.*

183. Donart, Gary B.

1969   Carbohydrate reserves of six mountain range plants as related to growth. *J. Range Mgmt.* 22(6):411-415.

Total available carbohydrates (mg/g) measured at various times during growing season.

Species: *Agropyron inerme, Stipa lettermanii, Symphoricarpos vaccinioides, Chrysothamnus viscidflorus, Senecio integerrimus,* and *Geranium fremontii.*

184. Donart, Gary B. and C. W. Cook

1970 Carbohydrates reserve content of mountain range plants following defoliation and regrowth. *J. Range Mgmt.* 23 (1):15-19.

Graphs showing quantity of carbohydrate regenerated: defoliation of grasses and forbes early in season (low CHO reserves) much more detrimental than defoliation late in season when reserves are high (providing there is time for regrowth before fall dormancy).

Species: *Agropyron inerme, Stipa lettermanii, Symphoricarpos vaccinioides, Chrysothamnus viscidflorus, Senecio integerrimus,* and *Geranium fremontii.*

185. Dorrell, D. G.

1971 Fatty acid composition of buckwheat seed. *J. Amer. Oil Chem. Soc.* 48(11):693-696.

Nutr. Abstr., 42:7977.

Species: *Fagopyrum sagittatum* (2 vars.), *F. tataricum;* also the wild form, *Polygonum convolvulus.*

186. Downs, A. A.

1944 Estimating acorn crops for wildlife in the southern Appalachians. *J. Wildl. Mgmt.* 8(4):339-340.

Number of acorns/lb., wt/100 acorns, average number of acorns/tree species and tree diameter per year. Also, average acorn crop/acre in Bent Creek Exp. Forest, North Carolina.

Species: Chestnut oak, white oak, eastern red oak, black oak and scarlet oak.

187. Downs, A. A. and W. E. McQuilkin

1944 Seed production of southern Appalachian oaks. *J. Forestry* 42(12):913-920.

188. Duell, R. W. and H. W. Guasman

1957 The effect of differential cutting on the yield, persistence protein, and mineral content of birdsfoot trefoil. *Agron. J.* 49:318-319.

Protein, P, K, Ca and yield.

Species: *Lotus corniculatus* L.

189. Duisberg, Peter C.

1952 Development of a feed from the creosote bush and the determination of its nutritive value. *J. Anim. Sci.* 11: 174-180.

Proximate analysis of both extracted and unextracted leaves (moisture-free); analysis on air-dry basis of extracted creosote feed for H_2O, Na, K, Ca, Mg, Fe, Cl, S, P, Ca/P, carotene (mg/lb), amino acids (Arg, Try, Phe, Leu, Ile, Val, Gly, Glu, Asp, Cys, Tyr), and coefficient of digestibility given. All data compared against alfalfa. Method: extraction of creosote from leaves with ethanol; residue is free of odor and bitter taste.

Species: *Larrea divaricata* Cav.

190. Duncan, D. A. and E. A. Epps, Jr.

1958 Minor mineral elements and other nutrients in forest ranges in Central Louisiana. La. Agr. Exp. Sta. *Bulletin,* 516.

191. Duncan, Wilbur H., P. L. Piercy and R. Starling

> 1955 Toxicological studies of southeastern plants. I. Leguminosae. *Econ. Bot.* 9(3):243-255.

192. Duncan, Wilbur H., P. L. Piercy, S. D. Feurt and R. Starling

> 1957 Toxicological studies of southeastern plants. II. Compositae. *Econ. Bot.* 11(1):75-85.

E

193. Earle, F. R.

> 1970 Epoxy oils from plant seeds. *J. Amer. Oil Chem. Soc.* 47(12):510-513.

194. Earle, F. R., A. S. Barclay and I. A. Wolff

> 1966 Compositional variation in seed oils of the *Crepis* genus. *Lipids* 1(2):325-327.

195. Earle, F. R., C. A. Glass, G. C. Geisinger, I. A. Wolff and Q. Jones

> 1960 Search for new industrial oils IV. *J. Amer. Oil Chem. Soc.* 37(9):440-447.

196. Earle, F. R., C. H. Van Etten, T. F. Clark and I. A. Wolff

> 1968 Compositional data on sunflower seed. *J. Amer. Oil Chem. Soc.* 45(12):876-879.

197. Earle, F. R., E. H. Melvin, L. H. Mason, C. H. Van Etten, I. A. Wolff and Q. Jones

1959   Search for new industrial oils I. Selected oils from 24 plant families. *J. Amer. Oil Chem. Soc.* 36(7):304-307.

198. Earle, F. R., I. A. Wolff, C. A. Glass and Q. Jones

1962   Search for new industrial oils VII. *J. Amer. Oil Chem. Soc.* 39(9):381-383.

199. Earle, F. R., I. A. Wolff and Q. Jones

1960   Search for new industrial oils III. Oils from Compositae. *J. Amer. Oil Chem. Soc.* 37(5):254-256.

200. Earle, F. R., K. L. Mikolajczak, I. A. Wolff and A. S. Barclay

1964   Search for new industrial oils X. Seed oils of the Calenduleae. *J. Amer. Oil Chem. Soc.* 41(5):345-347.

201. Earle, F. R. and Q. Jones

1962   Analysis of seed samples from 113 plant families. *Econ. Bot.* 16(4):221-250.

Analysis of more than 900 species of 501 genera in 113 families representing 35 orders of angiospermae and 2 orders of gymnospermae.

Percent ash, protein, oil, fraction N soluble in alcohol, fraction N soluble in trichloracetic acid, presence-absence data on starch, alkaloid and tannin tests, data on extracted oils: percent HBr-absorbing acid (as C_{18} acid), Halphen test, infrared analyses.

202. Earle, F. R., T. A. McGuire, J. Mallan, M. O. Bagby, I. A. Wolff and Q. Jones

> 1960 Search for new industrial oils II. Oils with high iodine values. *J. Amer. Oil Chem. Soc.* 37(1):48-50.

203. Edel 'stejn, M. M.

> 1968 Free amino acids in the seeds of some lupin species. *Dokl. Vses. Akad. Sel 'skokoz. Nauk* 2:13-14.
>
> Nutr. Abstr., 38:6751.

204. Edwards, D. W. and R. A. Goff

> 1935 Factors affecting the chemical composition of pasture grasses. Hawaii Agr. Exp. Sta. *Bulletin, 76.*

205. Edwards, H. M., Jr.

> 1964 Fatty acid composition of feeding stuffs. Georgia Agric. Exp. Sta. *Tech. Bulletin,* N.S. 36, June, 1964, pp. 34.
>
> Nutr. Abstr., 35:269.
>
> Thirty-two plant and animal feeds analyzed for fatty acid composition.

206. Ehlig, C. F., W. H. Allaway, E. E. Cary and J. Kubota

> 1968 Differences among plant species in selenium accumulation from soils low in available selenium. *Agron. J.* 60: 43-47.

207. Einarsen, Arthur S.

> 1946 Crude protein determination of deer food as an applied

Einarsen, Arthur S. (cont.)

management technique. *Trans. N. Amer. Wildl. Conf.* 11:309-312.

Percentage of protein by seasons for 6 browse species (shrubs of Oregon) and protein values (%) for 5 species (preferred deer foods) on old and newly-burned areas.

Species: Salmonberry, blackberry, thimbleberry, fireweed, vine maple, red alder, red elder, red huckleberry.

208. —.

1946 Management of black-tailed deer. *J. Wildl. Mgmt.* 10(1): 54-59.

Percent protein content for browse.

Species: *Acer circinatum* (vine maple), *Alnus rubra* (red alder), *Rubus spectabilis* (salmonberry), *Sambucus racemosa* (red elderberry), *Rubus parviflorus* (thimbleberry), and *Epilobium angustifolium* (fireweed).

209. Ekpenyong, T.

1969 Amino acid content of seeds of orchard crops. *J. Sci. Food Agric.* 20:608-610.

Nutr. Abstr., 40:2531.

210. Elvehjem, C. A. and W. H. Peterson

1928 The iron content of plant and animal food. *J. Biol. Chem.* 78:215-223.

Rather dated and of questionable use. Reports Fe and H_2O content of various plant and animal foods.

211. Engelter, Carola and A. S. Wehmeyer

1970   Fatty acid composition of oils of some edible seeds of wild plants. *J. Agri. Food Chem.* 18:25-26.

Five South African genera analyzed.

Species: *Sclerocarya, Bauhinia, Ricinodendron, Trichilia* and *Adansonia.*

212. Ernst, A. J., H. M. Sutcliffe and S. I. Aronovsky

1951   Agricultural residue pulps-*Crotolaria* pulps. *Tappi* 34(6): 247-251.

213. Errington, P. L.

1931   The bobwhite's winter food. *American Game* 20:November-December.

214. Esplin, A. C., J. E. Greaves and L. A. Stoddart

1937   A study of Utah ranges, composition of forage plants and use of supplements. Utah Agr. Exp. Sta. *Bulletin,* 277, 47 pp.

F

215. Farrar, W. V.

1966   Tecuitlatl; a glimpse of Aztec food technology. *Nature* 211, pp. 341-342.

The use of dried blue-green algae from the lake as a food resource.

216. Fashingbauer, B. A. and J. B. Moyle

1963 Nutritive value of red osier dogwood and mountain maple as deer browse. *Proc. Minnesota Acad. Sci.* 31(1):73-77.

Upper and lower portions of stems of red-osier dogwood compared for proximate contents, Ca, P and carotene with each other, mountain maple, alfalfa hay, red clover hay and timothy hay. Comparisons also made between mountain maple and red-osier dogwood on a month-by-month basis for 8 months of 1957-1958.

Species: *Cornus stolonifera, Acer spicatum.*

217. Fernandes, E. and M. B. Lira

1962 (Food value of cassava flours produced in Amazonas), *Arq. brasil Nutricao,* 18:87-94. Portuguese: English and French Summaries.

Nutr. Abstr., 34:5577.

Proximate contents, Ca, P, and Fe.

218. Finn, R. F.

1953 Foliar nitrogen and growth of certain mixed and pure forest plants. *J. Forestry* 51:31-33.

Various mixtures of 9 species of trees sampled at 4th, 6th, 10th and 12th years for mean height, diameter and *foliar nitrogen.* These are compared to see the effect of planting under different covers (black locust, shortleaf pine, old field and sassafras).

Species: *Liriodendron tulipfera* L., *Fraxinus pennsylvanica* var. *lanceolata* (Borkh.) Sarg., *Juniperus virginiana* L., *Acer saccharinum* L., *Liquidambar styraciflua* L., *Juglans nigra* L., *Quercus alba* L., *Q. rubra* L., black cherry.

219. Fisher, Harry J.

1947   Commercial feeding stuffs. Report on inspection 1946, Conn. Agr. Exp. Sta. *Bulletin*, No. 507, pp. 1-108, New Haven.

Proximate analyses of native grains, seeds, berries, etc.

220. Fleming, G. A.

1965   Trace elements in plants with particular reference to pasture species. *Outlook on Agriculture* 4:270-285.

221. Fletcher, K. and V. C. Brink

1969   Content of certain trace elements in range forages from South Central British Columbia. *Canad J. Plant Sci.* 49:517-520.

Nutr. Abstr., 40:2546.

Ppm dry matter: Cu, Mo, Pb, Zn, Se.

Species: *Astragalus serotinus* (timber milk vetch), *Arnica cordifolia* (arnica), *Calamagrostis rubescens* (pinegrass), *Poa pratensis* (Kentucky bluegrass), *Agropyron spicatum* (bluebunch wheatgrass): *Lupinus sericens* (Lupin).

222. Fletcher, Peter W. and J. Ochroymowych

1955   Mineral nutrition and growth of eastern and red cedar in Missouri. Missouri Agr. Exp. Sta. *Bulletin*, 577, 16 p.

Foliar P in seedlings and mature trees.

Species: *Juniperus virginiana* L.

Conclusion: Foliar P directly related to the concentration of soluble P in soil.

223. Flores, M., M. T. Menchu, M. Y. Lara and G. Arroyave

1969   Contenido de vitamina A en los alimentos incluidos en la tabla de composicion de alimentos para uso en America Latina. (Vitamin A in the foods included in the tables of composition of foods for Latin America.) *Arch. Latinoamer. Nutricion* 19:311-324.

Nutro. Abstr., 40:4851.

224. Forbes, E. B. and S. I. Bechdel

1931   Mountain laurel and rhododendron as foods for the white tailed deer. *Ecology* 12(2):323-333.

Rhododendron leaf, rhododendron bud and mountain laurel (leaf, bud and green stem taken together) analyzed for H_2O, Ash, crude protein, carbohydrate (fiber and N-Free Extract), and Fat. These analyses are compared to values for timothy hay (in seed).

Species: *Kalmia latifolia* (mountain laurel), *Rhododendron maximum* (Rhododendron).

225. —.

1935   The status of mountain laurel and rhododendron as foods for the white-tailed deer. Penn. Board of Game Commissions *Bulletin*, 12.

226. Forbes, R. M. and W. P. Garrigus

1950   Some effects of forage composition on its nutritive value when cut and fed green to steers and wethers, as determined conventionally and by the lignin ratio. *J. Anim. Sci.* 9:531-539.

Proximate contents, lignin, digestion coefficients and methoxyl content of lignin (determined from both

Forbes, R. M. and W. P. Garrigus (cont.)

forage and feces).

Species: Bluegrass, orchard grass, Ky. fescue, alfalfa, timothy, Lincoln brome, and ladino clover.

227. —.

1950   Some relationships between chemical composition, nutritive value, and intake of forage grazed by steers and wethers. *J. Anim. Sci.* 9(3):354-362.

Proximate contents and coefficients of digestibility (steers).

Species: Kentucky bromegrass, bluegrass, Ky. fescue, timothy hay, orchard grass, red top grass, ladino clover, Kenland red clover, Ky. 215 red clover, alfalfa, Lincoln bromegrass.

228. Fowells, Harry A. and R. W. Krauss

1959   The inorganic nutrition of Loblolly pine and Virginia pine with special reference to nitrogen and phosphorus. *For. Sci.* 5(1):95-112.

Top/root ratio (for N and P), change in height, total dry weight of seedling, N and P content (%) in dry material. Also, Ca, K, and Na (%) in foliage.

Sand-cultured seedlings analyzed for internal concentration of N and P after being given various rates in nutrient form.

Species: *Pinus taeda* L. and *P. virginiana* Mill.

229. Fraps, G. S. and J. F. Fudge

   1950   The chemical composition of forage grasses of the east
          Texas timber country. Texas Agr. Exp. Sta. *Bulletin,* No.
          582.

230. Fraps, George S.

   1919   Feeding values of certain feeding stuffs. Texas Agr. Exp.
          Sta. *Bulletin,* No. 245.

          Proximate analyses of various types of acorns, alfalfa,
          hay, beargrass (*Yucca glauca*), beet pulp, ground corn
          cobs, cotton burs, cotton seed, and peanut hulls are re-
          ported.

231. French, M. H.

   1957   Nutritional value of tropical grasses and fodders. *Herb.*
          Abstr. 27(1):1-9.

232. French, R. B.

   1962   Analysis of pecan oils by gas-liquid chromatography and
          ultra-violet spectrophotometry. *J. Am. Oil Chem.* 39:
          176-178.

233. Friedemann, W. G.

   1920   The carbohydrates of the pecan. *J. Am. Chem. Soc.*
          42(11):2286-2288.

          Analyses of *Carya olivaeformis.*

234. Fudge, J. F. and C. S. Fraps

   1944   The chemical composition of forage grasses from the Gulf

Fudge, J. F. and G. S. Fraps (cont.)

> Coast Prairie as related to soils and to requirements for range cattle. Texas Agric. Exp. Sta. *Bulletin*, No. 644.

235. —.

> 1945 The chemical composition of forage grasses from Northeast Texas a related to soils and to requirements for range cattle. Texas Agr. Exp. Sta. *Bulletin*, No. 776.

G

236. Gagnon, J. D.

> 1966 Free amino-acid content in needles of *Abies balsamea* and *Picea mariana* growing on different sites. *Nature* 212: 844.

237. Gastler, G. F., A. L. Moxon and W. T. McKean

> 1951 Composition of some plants eaten by deer in the Black Hills of South Dakota. *J. Wildl. Mgmt.* 15(4):352-357.

> Proximate contents, Ca, P, Fe and Mn.

> Species: *Populus tremuloides, Arctostaphylos uva-ursi, Amelanchier spicata, Juniperus communis, Rosa spinosissima, Ceanothus velutinus, Odostemon repens, Corylus rostrata, Poa* sp., *Shepherdia canadensis, Betula papyrifera, Pinus ponderosa, Juniperus horizontalis, Prunus melanocarpa, Quercus macrocarpa, Symphoricarpos occidentalis, Yucca glauca, Ostrya virginiana.*

238. Gawda, H. and M. Ralska

1965 (Role of herbs in supplying minerals and trace elements to animals. 2.) *Rocz, Nauk rol.* (B), 86:663-688. Polish: Russian and English summaries.

Nutr. Abstr., 36:5902.

Proximate components, Na, K, Ca, Mg, P, S, Si, Mn, Fe, Cu, Co and Mo. Many genera reported on are common to the Western Hemisphere.

239. Gentle, W., F. R. Humphreys and M. J. Lambert

1965 An examination of a *Pinus radiata* phosphate fertilizer trial fifteen years after treatment. *For. Sci.* 11(3):315-324.

Chemical analysis of foliage samples grouped by treatments—report of P, Al, Ca, Mg, K, Na, Fe, (ppm) content.

240. Gerhold, H. D.

1959 Seasonal variation of cholorplast pigments and nutrient elements in the needles of geographic races of Scotch pine. *Silvae Genet.* 8:105-123.

241. Gerloff, E. D., I. H. Lima and M. A. Stahmann

1965 Leaf proteins as foodstuffs. Amino acid composition of leaf protein concentrates. *J. Agric. Food Chem.* 12:139-143.

Nutr. Abstr., 35:5525.

Chenopodium, Nasturtium and various cultigens are analyzed.

242. Gerloff, G. C., D. D. Moore and J. T. Curtis

1964   Mineral content of native plants of Wisconsin. Univ. of Wisconsin Exp. Sta., College of Agr. Res. *Report* No. 14.

Analyses of more than 200 species for N, P, S. Ca, Mg, K, Fe, Cu, Zn, Mn, Mo, B, Cl, Sr, on a dry basis. Also tabulated for each specie are vegetative community, soil, pH, collection location, generic, specific and common names.

243. Gessel, S. P. and R. B. Walker

1956   Height growth response of Douglas-fir to nitrogen fertilization. *Proc. Amer. Soil Sci. Soc.* 20:97-100.

(N) in needles ranged from 0.91 percent in shallow gravelly soils to 2.1 percent in deep loam. In one experiment, nitrogen content of needles increased from 1.17 percent to 2.45 percent after 280 lbs. of ammonium nitrate and 320 lbs. of ammonium sulfate were applied per acre. N conc. of vigorous green foliage was 1.1-1.7 percent compared to 0.6-0.8 percent for yellow foliage.

244. Gilmore, A. R.

1972   Liming retards height growth of young shortleaf pine. *Soil Sci.* 113(6):448-452.

Analysis of foliar chemical elements N, P, K, Ca, Mg, Zn, B, Mn, Al correlated with heights of 5 year old shortleaf pines.

Species: *Pinus echinata* Mill.

245. Gladstones, J. S.

1962   The mineral composition of lupins. 2. A comparison of the copper, manganese, molybdenum and cobalt contents of lupins and other species at one site. *Austral. J. Exp.*

Gladstones, J. S. (cont.)

Agric. Animal Husb. 2:213-220.

Nutr. Abstr., 33:4167.

246. Goebel, Carl J. and C. W. Cook

1960 Effect of range condition on plant vigor, production and nutritive value of forage. *J. Range Mgmt.* 13(6):307-313.

Proximate analyses of 20 species sampled and compared according to range condition (poor vs. good); report of analyses of range plant composition, plant density, species productivity, lignin, cellulose, Ca, P contents and gross energy.

247. Goering, K. J., R. Eslick and D. C. Brelsford

1965 The composition of the oil of *Berteroa incana* and the potential value of its seed as a cash crop for Montana. *Econ. Bot.* 19(1):44-45.

248. —.

1965 A search for high erucic acid containing oils in the Cruciferae. *Econ. Bot.* 19(3):251-256.

249. Gomez, E.

1967 (The stem of the banana plant as a food for man. Preliminary communication.) *Rev. Fac. Farm Biogum.,* Sao Paulo 5:259-268.

Nutr. Abstr., 40:2536.

Proximate analyses, Mn, P, Ca, Na, Fe and K.

Species: *Musa cavendishi* Lamb.

250. Gomez-brenes, R. A., L. G. Elias and R. Bressani

1968   (Effect of ripening of maize on its nutritive value.) *Arch. Latinoamer. Nutricion* 18:65-79. Spanish: English Summary.

Nutr. Abstr., 39:292.

Proximate and amino acid components reported. Study of maize at different stages during its developmental cycle.

251. Gomide, J. A.

1968   Nutritive evaluation of six tropical grasses grown in Central Brazil. *Dissertation Abstrts.* (B) 29:822B-823B.

Nutr. Abstr., 39:4626.

Some proximate components.

Species: Molasses (*Melinis minutiflora*), pangola (*Digitaria decumbens*), Kikuyu (*Pennisetum clandestinum*), Napier (*P. purpureum*), Suwanee Bermuda (*Cynodon dactylon*), Sempre verde grass.

252. Gomide, J. A., C. H. Noller, G. O. Moh, J. H. Conrad and D. L. Hill

1969   Mineral composition of six tropical grasses as influenced by plant age and nitrogen fertilization. *Agronomy J.* 61:120-123.

Nutr. Abstr., 40:299.

K, P, Ca, Mg, Cu, Mn, Fe and Zn contents.

Species from Central Brazil.

68

253. Goodall, D. W. and F. G. Gregory

1947   Chemical composition of plants as an index of their nutritional status. Imp. Bur. Hort. and Plantation Crops. East Malling, Kent, England. *Tech. Communications,* 17:167.

Prime reference for the use of foliar analysis as a guide to the nutritional requirements of plants.

254. Goodall, H.

1969   The composition of fruits. B.F.M.I.R.A. *Sci. Tech. Surveys,* September, 1969. No. 59, pp. 101.

Nutr. Abstr., 40:7101.

197 references. Literature mainly since 1950 tabulated for soluble, insoluble, and total solids, acidity as citric acid, ash, ash alkalinity, Na, K, Ca, Mg, P, N, formol number, chloramine value, amino acids, flavenoids and polyphenols. See abstract for list of fruits—mostly popular western types.

255. Goodrum, P. D., U. H. Reid and C. E. Boyd

1971   Acorn yields, characteristics and management criteria of oaks for wildlife. *J. Wildl. Mgmt.* 35(3):520-532.

Species: *Quercus prinus, Q. alba, Q. stellata, Q. marilandica, Q. nigra, Q. cinerea, Q. falcata, Q. lyrata, Q. virginiana, Q. phellos.*

256. Goodrum, Phil D.

1959   Acorns in the diet of wild life. *Proceedings of the 13th annual conference S. E. Assoc. Game and Fish Commissioners, 1959, Baltimore, Maryland,* pp. 54-61.

Goodrum, Phil D. (cont.)

> Proximate analyses of various species, yields/trees and acorn requirements of some animals/day.

257. Gordon, Aaron and A. W. Sampson

> 1939 Composition of common California foothill plants as a factor in range management. Calif. Agr. Exp. Sta. *Bulletin*, 627, 95 pp.

> Proximate contents, Ca, P and K.

258. Greene, R. A.

> 1936 The composition and the uses of the fruit of the giant cactus (Carnegia gigantea) and its products. *J. Chem. Educ.* 13:309-312.

> Proximate analyses of native Arizona plants.

> Species: *Opuntia* sp., *Agave parryi, Cereus giganteus (Carnegia gigantea), Prosopis juliflora, Salvia columbariae, Sysimbrium pinnatum (Sophia pinnata)* and *Yucca arizonica.*

> Also some information provided on methods of food preparation.

259. Greenwood, E. A. N. and E. G. Hallsworth

> 1960 Studies on the nutrition of forage legumes. II. Some interactions of calcium, phosphorous, copper and molybdenum on the growth and chemical composition of *Trifolium subterraneum* L. *Plant and Soil* XII(2):97-128.

260. Gross, A. T. H. and B. R. Stefansson

1966   Effect of planting date on protein, oil and fatty acid content of rape seed and turnip rape. *Canad. J. Plant Sci.* 46:389-395.

Nutr. Abstr., 37:304.

261. Grotelueschen, R. D. and D. Smith

1967   Determination and identification of non-structural carbohydrates removed from grass and legume tissue by various sulfuric acid concentrations, taka diastase, and water. *J. Agric. Food Chem.* 15(6):1048-1051.

Nutr. Abstr., 38:4517.

Determination of raffinose, maltose, sucrose, glucose, fructose, mannose, galactose, arabinose and xylose (percent dry wt.) for timothy and alfalfa.

262. Grove, M. D., M. E. Daxenbichler, D. Weisleder and C. H. VanEtten

1971   The structure of pinnatanine, a new amino acid amide from *Staphylea pinnata* L. *Tetrahedron Lett.* 47:4477-4480.

Pinnatanine: 3 percent yield from defatted seed meal of *Staphylea pinnata* L. (European bladdernut, Staphyleaceae); also found in *Hemerocallis fulva* L. (common orange day lily, Liliaceae).

263. Gunstone, F. D., D. Kilcast, R. G. Powell and G. M. Taylor

1967   *Afzelia cuanzensis* seed oil: a source of crepenynic and 14, 15-dehydrocrepenynic acid. *Chem. Commun.* (6): 295-296.

264. Gunstone, F. D., G. M. Taylor, J. A. Cornelius and T. W. Hammonds

1968 New tropical seed oils II. Component aicds of leguminous and other seed oils. *J. Sci. Food Agri.* 19:706-709.

265. Gunstone, F. D., S. R. Steward, J. A. Cornelius and T. W. Hammonds

1972 New tropical seed oils. IV. Component acids of leguminous and other seed oils including useful sources of crepenynic and dehydrocrepenynic acid. *J. Sci. Food Agri.* 23: 53-70.

266. Gunther, F., O. Burckhart and I. Oostinga

1968 (Mineral contents of spices.) *Nutritio et Dieta* 10:151-160. German: English and French summaries.

Nutr. Abstr., 39:276.

Places of origin, culinary form, Mn, Fe, Cu, K, Na and Cl contents. Different portions of the plant have different mineral content, with leaves possessing the highest content.

267. Gupta, U. C., F. W. Calder and L. B. Macleod

1971 Influence of added limestone and fertilizers upon the micro-nutrient content of forage tissue and soil. *Plant and Soil* 35(2):249-256.

Nutr. Abstr., 42:5364.

Effects of pH and season on the uptake and availability of Mo, Cu, B, Mn and Zn in various forages.

268. Gurchinoff, Steve and W. L. Robinson

1972   Chemical characteristics of jackpine needles selected by feeding spruce grouse. *J. Wildl. Mgmt.* 36(1):80-87.

Proximate composition.

269. Gysel, L. W.

1956   Measurements of acorn crops. *Forest Sci.* 2(4):305-313.

A review of crop measurement techniques and a summary of factors affecting production: climate, age, crown exposure, individual variability (tabulated), environmental factors. An extensive bibliography is included.

270. Gysel, Leslie W.

1971   A 10-year analysis of beechnut production and use in Michigan. *J. Wildl. Mgmt.* 35(3):516-519.

H

271. Haas, A. R. C. and L. D. Batchelor

1928   Relation of phosphorous content to shriveling of walnut kernels. *Botanical Gazette* 86(4):448-455. Chicago.

272. Habib, A. A.

1973   A new sesquiterpene keto-lactone from *Senecio*. *Planta Med.* 23:88-93.

273. Hagemann, J. M., F. R. Earle, I. A. Wolff and A. S. Barclay

1967 Search for new industrial oils. XIV. Seed oils of Labiatae. *Lipids* 2(5):371-380.

274. Hagan, H. L.

1953 Nutritive value for deer of some forage plants in the Sierra Nevada, Calif. *Fish and Game* 39(2):163-175.

Proximate analyses of oven-dry samples of 13 species of forage plants.

Species: *Ceanothus cuneatus, Chamaebatia foliolosa, Ceanothus integerrimus, Cercocarpus betuloides, Arctostaphylos patula, A. mariposa, Ceanothus cordulatus, Prunus emarginata, Ceanothus prostratus, C. velutinus, Amelanchier alnifolia, A. patula, Purshia tridentata.*

275. Halls, L. K., O. M. Hale and F. G. Know

1957 Seasonal variation in grazing use, nutritive content, and digestibility of wiregrass forage. Ga. Agr. Exp. Sta. *Bulletin*, N.S. II, 28 pp.

276. Halls, L. K. and R. Alcaniz

1968 Browse plants yield best in forest openings. *J. Wildl. Mgmt.* 32(1):185-186.

Fruit and forage yields compared for plants growing in open areas and under forest. Those in open clearings average 32 times more fruit and 7 times more twig growth.

Species: *Ilex vomitoria, Callicarpa americana, Lonicera japonica, Berchemia scandens, Euonymus americanus, Cornus florida, Gelsemium sempervirens.*

74

277. Hamilton, J. W. and C. S. Gilbert

1966   Composition of three species of *Vaccinium. Advancing Frontiers Plant Sci.* 17:71-80.

        Nutr. Abstr., 39:6709.

        Carotene, energy, proximate analysis, Ca, P, K, Mg, S, Co, Cu, Mn, Fe, Mo of vegetative terminal portions.

        Species: Wyoming specimens of *Vaccinium scoparium* Leiberg, *V. caespitosum* Michx., *V. membranaceum* Dougl. exHook.

278. —.

1968   Comparative mineral composition of longstalk and alsike clovers. *J. Range Mgmt.* 21(1):53-55.

        Ca, P, Mg, Na, K, S, Fe, Mn, Mo, Cu, Co, Zn, contents. Longstalk is native, alsike an introduced clover.

279. —.

1971   Mineral composition of native and introduced clovers. *J. Range Mgmt.* 24(4):304-308.

        Percentage Ca, P, Mg, Na, K and S; ppm Co, Cu, Fe, Mn, Mo and Zn. Oven-dry weight.

        Species: Seven native and 4 introduced clovers collected from widely scattered areas of Wyoming and southern Montana.

280. Hamilton, John W.

1961   Native clovers and their chemical composition. *J. Range Mgmt.* 14(6):327-331.

Hamilton, John W. (cont.)

> Proximate analyses plus Ca, P, Mg of 7 species. Most sampled in bloom stage (2 in seed stage).

281. Hamilton, John W. and O. A. Beath

> 1963 Uptake of available selenium by certain range plants. *J. Range Mgmt.* 16(5):261-265.
>
> For 20 types of plants the total, soluble, soluble inorganic, soluble organic and insoluble quantities (ppm) of selenium are reported. Method: A known Se concentration is added to Se-free greenhouse soil, plants are grown from seed and are later analyzed.

282. Harshbarger, Thomas J. and B. S. McGinnes

> 1971 Nutritive value of sourwood leaves. *J. Wildl. Mgmt.* 35 (4):668-673.
>
> Nutr. Abstr., 42:8020.
>
> Ca, P, K, Fe, Na, Mn, Cu, Proximate components. A comparison is made between green and dead leaves.
>
> Species: *Oxydendrum arboreum.*

283. Hart, G. H., H. R. Guilbert and H. Goss

> 1932 Seasonal changes in the chemical composition of range forage and their relation to nutrition of animals. Calif. Agr. Exp. Sta. *Bulletin,* 543, 62 pp.

284. —.

> 1932 Seasonal changes in the chemical composition of range forage and their relation to nutrition of animals. Calif. Agr. Exp. Sta. *Bulletin,* 600, 50 pp.

285. Harvey, D.

Tables of the amino acids in foods and feedstuffs, Commonwealth Bur. Animal Nutrition *Tech. Commun.* No. 19, 2nd Ed., 1970, pp. v + 105. [Obtainable from Commonwealth Agric. Bur., Farham Royal, Slough, Bucks.]

Up to 18 amino acids on 1,918 samples.

286. Hatch, Carl F.

1968 Chemical composition and nylon bag digestibility of range grasses. Unpubl. M.S. thesis. New Mexico State Univ., Las Cruces, 71 pp.

287. Hawf, L. R. and W. E. Schmid

1967 Uptake and translocation of zinc by intact plants. *Plant and Soil* 27:249-260.

Competitive effects of Zn, Cu, and Mn on translocation in tops and roots of plants.

288. Hawkins, G. E.

1959 Relationships between chemical composition and some nutritive qualities of *Lespedeza sericea* Hays. *J. Anim. Sci.* 18(2):763-769.

Proximate contents, lignin, cellulose, tannin and other carbohydrates.

289. Heady, H. F., D. W. Cooper, J. M. Rible and J. F. Hooper

1963 Comparative forage values of California oatgrass and soft chess. *J. Range Mgmt.* 16:51-54.

Crude protein, crude fiber and P (annual cycle).

77

Heady, H. F., D. W. Cooper, J. M. Rible and J. F. Hooper
(cont.)

Species: *Danthonia californica, Bromus mollis.*

290. Hedrick, D. W., J. A. B. McArthur, J. E. Oldfield and J. A.
Young

1965 Seasonal yield and chemical content of forage mixtures
on a pine woodland meadow site in Northeastern Oregon.
Oregon Agri. Exp. Sta. *Tech. Bulletin,* 84, June 5, 42 pp.
1965.

Nutr. Abstr., 36:5890.

291. Heinze, Ph. H and A. E. Murneek

1940 Comparative accuracy and efficiency in determination of
carbohydrates in plant material. Mo. Agr. Exp. Sta. *Res.
Bulletin,* 314, 23 pp.

292. Hellmes, Henry

1940 A study of monthly variations in the nutritive value of
several natural winter deer foods. *J. Wildl. Mgmt.* 4(3):
315-325.

Proximate analysis on monthly basis (November-April) of
shoots from the previous growing season.

Species: *Corylus americanus, Acer rubrum, Cornus
paniculata, Salix humilis, Populus tremuloides, Myrica
asplenifolia, Quercus ilicifolia, Q. prinoides.*

Marked differences found, esp. in N-free extract, protein,
and crude fiber, all of which exhibited trends indicating
reduction in nutritive value through the winter.

293. Herting, D. C. and E. J. E. Drury

1963 Vitamin E content of vegetable oils and fats. *J. Nutrition* 81:335-342.

Nutr. Abstr., 34:3939.

Values for total tocopherol and alpha-tocopherol are tabulated and presence of other tocopherols is noted for 38 fats or oils from seed of 17 plant species.

294. Hibbs, J. W. and M. W. Evans

1950 A comparison of the carotene content of different varieties of timothy harvested at various stages of development. *Agron. J.* 42(2):94-95.

295. Hilditch, T. P.

1956 The chemical constitution of natural fats, 3rd Ed., Wiley, New York.

296. Hill, A. C., S. J. Toth and F. E. Bear

1953 Cobalt status of New Jersey soils and forage plants and factors affecting the cobalt content of plants. *Soil Sci.* 76:273-284.

Minimum, maximum and average Co content of 9 species of weed, 9 vegetables, 5 cereals, 4 grasses and 6 legumes.

297. Hill, Douglas C., E. V. Evans and H. G. Lumsden

1968 Metabolizable energy of aspen flower buds for captive ruffed grouse. *J. Wildl. Mgmt.* 32(4):854-858.

Species: *Populus tremuloides.*

298. Hodges, John D., S. J. Barras and J. K. Mauldin

1968 Free and protein-bound amino acids in inner bark of loblolly pine. *For. Sci.* 14(3):330-333.

299. Hoehne, O. E.

1966 Cattle preference as related to chemical components of native range plants. Ph.D. thesis, Univ. of Nebraska, 137 pp.

300. Hoehne, O. E., D. C. Clanton and C. L. Streeter

1968 Chemical composition and *in vitro* digestibility of forbs consumed by cattle grazing native range. *J. Range Mgmt.* 21(1):5-7.

Species: *Tradescantia bracheata, Lappula redowski, Helianthus petiolaris, Lygodesmia rostrata, Yucca glauca, Chenopodium album, Artemisia filifolia.*

301. Hoffmann, R. S.

1961 The quality of the winter food of the blue grouse. *J. Wildl. Mgmt.* 25(2):209-210.

Crude protein content of white fir needles (*Abies concolor*), high crown needle content plotted separate from low crown needles for each month of a 3-year period.

302. Holgate, K. C.

1950 Changes in the composition of maple sap during the tapping season. N.Y. Agr. Exp. Sta. *Bulletin,* 742, Geneva, N.Y.

303. Holt, D. A. and A. R. Hilst

1969 Daily variation in carbohydrate content of selected forage crops. *Agronomy J.* 61:239-242.

Nutr. Abstr., 40:2549.

Species: *Medicago sativa, Poa pratensis, Bromus inermis, Festuca arundinacea.*

304. Holtz, H. E.

1930 Effect of calcium and phosphorous content of various soil series in Western Washington upon the calcium and phosphorous composition of oats, red clover and white clover. Wash. Agr. Exp. Sta. *Bulletin,* 243.

305. Hooker, H. D., Jr.

1920 Seasonal changes in the chemical composition of apple spurs. Mo. Agr. Exp. Sta. *Res. Bulletin,* 40, 51 pp.

306. Hopkins, C. Y. and M. J. Chisholm

1953 Some fatty acids of peanut, hickory and acorn oils. *Canad. J. Chem.* 31:1173-1180.

Nutr. Abstr. Rev., 24(3):522.

307. Hopper, T. H. and L. L. Nesbitt

1930 The chemical composition of some North Dakota pasture and haygrasses. N. Dak. Agr. Exp. Sta. *Bulletin,* 236, 39 pp.

308. Horwitt, M. K., G. R. Cowgill and L. B. Mendel

1936   The availability of the proteins and inorganic salts of the green leaf. *J. Nutr.* 12:237-254.

Tabulation of percentage tot. amino N liberated from spinach and casein by pepsin, trypsin and erepsin (1-336 hr. samples). Also, tabulation of availability of inorganic constituents of spinach as estimated by *in vitro* digestion trials.

309. Hough, Walter A.

1968   Carbohydrate reserves of saw-palmetto: seasonal variation and effects of burning. *Forest Sci.* 14(4):399-405.

Monthly carbohydrate content (%): total available carbohydrates, starch, reducing sugars, sucrose, and monthly moisture content (%) for burned and unburned plants.

Species: *Serenoa repens* (Bartr.) Small.

Periodic burning results in an increase in cellular activity which can be seen in the increase in moisture content and the conversion of a large quantity of the plants' starch reserves to sugar.

310. Hoyle, M. C.

1969   Response of yellow birch in acid subsoil to macronutrient additions. *Soil Sci.* 108(5):354-358.

Analyses of leaves, stems and roots to gauge effect of nutrient treatments on N, P, K, Ca, Mg, Mn, Al.

Species: *Betula alleghaniensis* Britton.

311. Huff, D. E.

1970 A study of selected nutrients in browse available to the ruffed grouse. M.S. Thesis, University of Minnesota, 72 pp.

A study of vegetative and flower buds of aspen.

312. Hundley, L. R.

1959 Available nutrients in selected deer-browse species growing on different soils. *J. Wildl. Mgmt.* 23(1):81-90.

Proximate analyses over 8 months at monthly intervals.

Species: *Cornus florida, Robinia pseudoacacia, Acer rubrum,* also *Pyrularia pubera, Rhododendron nudiflorum* and *R. calendulareum.*

313. Hungerford, K. E.

1957 Evaluating ruffed grouse foods for habitat improvement. *Trans. N. Am. Wildl. Conf.* 22:380-395.

Phenology of 16 species.

314. Hunter, H. H. and H. E. Hammar

1956 Relation of oil contents of pecan kernels to chemical components of leaves as a measure of nutrient status. *Soil Sci.* 82(4):261-269.

The N, P, K, Ca and Mg of leaves (milli-equivalents/100 gms of leaves) compared to the oil in kernels.

315. Hurwitz, Charles and K. C. Beeson

1944 Cobalt content of some food plants. *Food Res.* 9:348-357.

I

316. Idaho Agricultural Experimental Station

1937 Preliminary report on the composition of range forage plants as related to animal nutrition. Idaho Exp. Sta. *Mimeo Leaflet* 13, 23 pp.

317. Illinois Agricultural Experimental Station

1935 Nuts fail as adequate protein substitutes for meat. *Annual Report* 47:80-82.

318. Ingestad, T.

1957 Studies on the nutrition of forest tree seedlings. I. Mineral nutrition of birch. *Physiol. Plant.* 10:418-439.

Seedlings grown in nutrient solutions with various concentrations of N, P, K, Ca, Mg, S and Fe analyzed for mineral content. Leaves and roots analyzed separately.

319. —.

1959 Studies on the nutrition of forest tree seedlings. II. Mineral nutrition of spruce. *Physiol. Plant.* 12:568.

320. —.

1960 Studies on the nutrition of forest tree seedlings. III. Mineral nutrition of pine. *Physiol. Plant.* 13:513-533.

Ingestad, T. (cont.)

N, K, Mg, Ca, S, P, Fe mineral content analyses of needles, roots of seedlings grown in cultures of varying mineral content. Levels of element content corresponding to deficiency given for *Pinus sylvestris, P. strobus, P. resinosa, P. banksiana, P. taeda, P. virginiana, P. nigra, Picea, Abies, Betula verrucosa;* also levels corresponding to max. growth for these are reported.

J

321. Jackson, G. C.

1963   Ascorbic acid content of some *Malpighia* spp. *J. Agric. Univ. Puerto Rico* 47:201-204.

Nutr. Abstr., 34:2337.

Species: *Malpighia shaferi, M. infestissima, M. linearis, M. coccigera, M. suberosa.* 47 references to the above species and others.

322. Jaffe, W. G.

1968   Factores toxicos en leguminosas. [Toxic factors in legumes]. *Arch. latinoamer. Nutricion* 18:205-218. Spanish: English Summary.

Nutr. Abstr., 39:4591.

323. Jaffe, W. G., F. Wagner, P. Marcano and R. Hernandez

1964   [A toxic lipoglycoprotein fraction from *Ricinus communis*]. *Acta cientif. venezol.* 15:29-32. Spanish:

Jaffe, W. G., F. Wagner, P. Marcano and R. Hernandez (cont.)

English Summary.

Nutr. Abstr., 35:1942.

324. Jaffe, W. G., J. F. Chavez and M. C. de Mondragon

1967 [Se in Venezuelan foods]. *Arch. latinoamer. Nutricion* 17:59-68. Spanish: English Summary.

Nutr. Abstr., 38:273.

Data on primarily commercially produced foods, but reference includes *Lecythis ollaria* (in 2 samples of this species, Se reached 5100 and 8100 ppm).

325. —.

1969 Contenido de selenio en muestras de semilla de ajon-joli (*Sesamum indicum*) procedentes de varios paises. [Se content in samples of sesame seed (*Sesamum indicum*) from several countries]. *Arch. latinoamer. Nutricion* 19:299-307. Spanish: English Summary.

Nutr. Abstr., 40:4786.

326. Jakimov, A. P.

1965 [Composition of perennial Polygonaceae]. *Vestn. sel'-skoboz. Nauki.* 4:78-80. Russian.

Nutr. Abstr., 35:5561.

K, Ca, P, proximate components.

Species: *Polygonum weyrichii, P. sachalinense, P. div-aricatum.*

327. James, L. F., et al.

    1972   Estrogenic properties of locoweed (*Astragalus lenti-ginosus*). *Canad. J. Comp. Med.* 36:360-365.

328. Janicki, J., E. Sobkowska, J. Warchalewski, K. Nowakow-ska, J. Chelkowski and B. Stasinska

    1973   Amino acid composition of cereal and oilseed. *Die Nahrung* 17:359-365.

           Quantative analyses performed on hulled grain.

           Species: Millet, wheat, barley, rye, oats, buckwheat, sunflower, poppy seed, soybean and rapeseed.

329. Jart, A.

    1963   The fatty acid composition of filbert oil. *Acta Chem. Scand.* 17:1186-1187.

           Nutr. Abstr., 34:278.

           Species: *Corylus avellana*, grown in Denmark.

330. Jentsch, M. S. and A. F. Morgan

    1949   Thiamin, Riboflavin and Niacin content of walnuts. *Food Res.* 14:40-53.

331. Johnson, J. R. and J. T. Nichols

    1969   Crude protein content of eleven grasses as affected by yearly variation, legume association, and fertilization. *Agronomy J.* 61:65-68.

           Nutr. Abstr., 39:6716.

332. Johnson, June M. and G. W. Butler

1957 Iodine content of pasture plants. I. Method of determination and preliminary investigation of species and strain differences. *Physiol. Plantarum* 10:100-111.

Bibliography (24 references) Three reporting effect of species and season on herbage iodine content for 6 genera (10 species). ug/100g dry weight.

333. Johnston, A. and L. M. Bezeau

1962 Chemical composition of range forage plants of the *Festuca scabrella* association. *Canad. J. Plant Sci.* 42: 105-115.

Twenty grasses (5 stages of growth) and 10 herbaceous and shrubby species (at 3 stages of growth) analyzed for crude protein, crude fat, crude fiber, ash, Ca, P and carotene.

334. Johnston, A., L. M. Bezeau and S. Smoliak

1967 Variation in silica content of range grasses. *Canad. J. Plant Sci.* 47:65-71.

Nutr. Abstr., 37:6098.

Variation with respect to time and location and stage of growth.

Species: *Festuca scabrella, Stipa comata, Bouteloua gracilis, Carex filifolia, Deschampsia caespitosa.*

335. —.

1968 Chemical composition and *in vitro* digestibility of Alpine tundra plants. *J. Wildl. Mgmt.* 32(4):733-777.

Johnston, A., L. M. Bezeau and S. Smoliak (cont.)

> Crude protein, Ca, P, ash, silica, cellulose, coefficient of digestibility of cellulose.
>
> Species: *Agropyron latiglume, Bromus pumpellianus, Festuca brachyphylla, Festuca scabrella, Poa alpina, Carex scirpoidea, Luzula spicata, Epilobium angustifolium, Hedysarum sulphurescens, Pedicularis groenlandica, Phacelia lyall, Rumex alpestris, Senecio* spp., *S. triangularis, Thalictrum occidentale, Valeriana sitchensis, Potentilla fruticosa, Salix artica, Vaccinium caespitosum.*

336. Jones, Q. and F. R. Earle

> 1966   Chemical analyses of seeds II: Oil and protein content of 759 species. *Econ. Bot.* 20(2):127-155.
>
> Data on component analyzed; percent protein, percent oil, wt./1000 seeds; starch, alkaloid and tannin tests; data on extracted oil: HBr-absorbing acid, (as C_{18} acid), Halphen test, Infrared analysis.
>
> Bibliography contains 39 references.
>
> Species: 32 orders, 103 families, 465 genera, 759 species.

337. Jordan, J. V.

> 1955   Protein and mineral content of forage legumes and grasses in Idaho. Univ. Idaho Agr. Exp. Sta. *Bulletin,* 245, pp. 1-8.

338. Jung, G. A., B. Lilly, S. C. Shih and R. L. Reid

> 1964   Studies with sudangrass. I. Effect of growth stage and level of nitrogen fertilizer upon yield of dry matter; estimated digestibility of energy, dry matter and protein;

Jung, G. A., B. Lilly, S. C. Shih and R. L. Reid (cont.)

amino acid composition; and prussic acid potential. *Agron. J.* 56:533-537.

K

339. Kamstra, L. D., A. L. Moxon and O. G. Bentley

1958 The effect of stage of maturity and lignification on the digestion of cellulose in forage plants by rumen microorganisms *in vitro. J. Anim. Sci.* 17:199.

340. Kamstra, L. D., D. L. Schentzel, J. K. Lewis and R. L. Elderkin

1968 Maturity Studies with Western wheatgrass. *J. Range Mgmt.* 21(4):235-239.

In vitro cellulose digestion (%), at various cutting dates as well as respective levels of holocellulose, hemicellulose, cellulose, lignin, ash and protein (June-September) neutral sugars are also listed (xylose, arabinose, glucose, galactose-percent hemicellulose hydrolysate).

Species: *Agropyron smithii* Rydb.

341. Kamstra, L. D., R. W. Stanley and S. M. Ishizaki

1966 Seasonal and growth period changes of some nutritive components of kikuyu grass. *J. Range Mgmt.* 19(5):288-291.

Comparison of content of crude fiber, detergent fiber, cellulose, holocellulose, hemicellulose, percent dry basis

90

Kamstra, L. D., R. W. Stanley and S. M. Ishizaki (cont.)

for 4-10 week growth period (February-April). Also reported are lignin* and crude protein content.

*lignin— a) 72 percent sulfuric acid lignin
b) acid detergent lignin

342. Karetnikov, P. V. and M. M. Dimitricenko

1966 [Some trace elements in pine nuts]. *Vop. Pitan* 25(5): 79-80. Russian.

Nutr. Abstr., 37:2334.

mg/kg dry matter of I, Mn, Co, Cu, and Ni.

343. Kiesling, H. E., A. B. Nelson and C. H. Herbel

1969 Chemical composition of Tobosa grass collected by hand-plucking and esophageal-fistulated steers. *J. Range Mgmt.* 22(3):155-159.

Proximate composition.

Species: *Hilaria mutica* (Buckl.), Benth., and alfalfa.

344. Kik, M. C. and R. D. Staten

1957 The nutrient content of fescue and orchard grass and amino acids in other grassland species. *Agron. J.* 49: 248-250.

Proximate contents, lignin, Fe (total and available), P, K, carotene, P-aminobenzoic acid, choline, inositol, pyridoxine, folic acid (total and free), nicotinic acid, riboflavin, and thiamine in *Festuca arundinaceae,* and *Dactylis glomerata* (both in early hay). Also reported— amino acid content (17 amino acids) of 22 herbage plants.

91

Kik, M. C. and R. D. Staten (cont.)

Species: *Festuca arundinaceae, Dactylis glomerata, Sorghum vulgare* var. *Sudanensis* (6 registered strains), *Trifolium incarnatum* (5 registered strains), *Melilotus officinalis, M. albus, Medicago sativa* (2 strains), *Andropogon scoparius, A. gerardi, Bromus secalinus, Eragrostis curvula, Phalaris arundinaceae* and *Bromus inermis.*

345. Kilmer, V. J., O. L. Bennett, V. F. Stahly and D. R. Timmons

1960 Yield and mineral composition of eight forage species grown in four levels of soil moisture. *Agron. J.* 52(5): 282-285.

Percent N, P, K, Ca, Mg, S, ppm B, Mn, Fe, Al, Cu, for 4 moisture levels. Relative total uptake of ions by plants grown at 4 moisture levels. Comparison of effect of 3 moisture levels on weight of roots and total amount of each element in the tops of forage species (lb./acre).

Species: Two alfalfa varieties, 3 types of clover and 3 species of grass.

346. King, T. R. and H. W. Titus

1943 Acorns of the willow oak, *Quercus phellos,* a source of vitamin A activity. *Poultry Sci.* 22(1):56-60.

347. King, Thomas R. and H. E. McClure

1944 Chemical composition of some American wild feedstuffs. *J. of Agri. Res.* 69(1):33-46. Washington.

Proximate analysis of feedstuffs for domestic animals.

Species: Ten genera of legume seeds; 7 genera of gramineae (grass) seeds; 5 genera of misc. families of seed

King, Thomas R. and H. E. McClure (cont.)

> plants, 4 genera of mast trees (*Quercus, Corylus, Pinus* and *Liquidambar*); 17 genera of various families of fruit plants (12 families) and 1 species of *Cyperus*.

348. Kinsella, J. E.

> 1970 Evaluation of plant leaf protein as a source of food protein. *Chem. Indust.* pp. 550-554.
>
> A review with 41 references.

349. Kinsinger, Floyd E. and H. H. Hopkins

> 1961 Carbohydrate content of underground parts of grasses as affected by clipping. *J. Range Mgmt.* 14(1):9-12.
>
> Percent total readily available carbohydrate and hemicellulose in control, moderately clipped and heavily clipped samples taken over a 2 year period.
>
> Species: *Andropogon gerardi* Vitmani, *Agropyron smithii* Rydb. *Bouteloua gracilis* (H.B.K.) Lag ex Stend., *Buchloe dactyloides* (Nutt.) Engelm.

350. Kleiman, R., C. R. Smith, Jr., S. G. Yates and Q. Jones

> 1965 Search for new industrial oils. XII. Fifty-eight Euphorbiaceae oils, including one rich in vernolic acid. *J. Amer. Oil Chemists Soc.* 42(3):169-172.

351. Kleiman, R., F. R. Earle and I. A. Wolff

> 1966 The *Trans-3-enoic* acids of *Grindelia oxylepis* seed oil. *Lipids* 1(2):301-304.

352. Kleiman, R., F. R. Earle and I. A. Wolff

    1969   Dihydrosterculic acid, a major fatty acid component of *Euphoria longana* seed oil. *Lipids* 4(5):317-320.

353. —.

    1969   Wax esters from sunflower tank settlings. *J. Amer. Oil Chemists Soc.* 46(9):505.

354. Kleiman, R., F. R. Earle, I. A. Wolff and Q. Jones

    1964   Search for new industrial oils. XI. Oils of Boraginaceae. *J. Amer. Oil Chemists Soc.* 41(7):459-460.

355. —.

    1968   Addendum: search for industril oils XI. Oils of Boraginaceae. *J. Amer. Oil Chemists Soc.* 45(5):408.

356. Kleiman, R. and G. F. Spencer

    1971   Ricinoleic acid in *Linum mucronatum* seed oil. *Lipids* 6(12):962-963.

357. Kleiman, R., G. F. Spencer, F. R. Earle, H. J. Nieschlag and A. S. Barclay

    1972   Tetra-acid triglycerides containing a new hydroxy eicosadienoyl moiety in *Lesquerella auriculata* seed oil. *Lipids* 7(10):660-665.

358. Kleiman, R., G. F. Spencer, F. R. Earle and I. A. Wolff

    1967   Fatty acid composition of *Ephedra campylopoda* oil. *Chem. Ind.* 31:1326-1327.

359. Kleiman, R., G. F. Spencer, L. W. Tjarks and F. R. Earle

1971 Oxygenated *Trans*-3-olefinic acids in a Stenachaenium seed oil. *Lipids* 6(8):617-622.

Species: *Stenachaenium macrocephalum* (Compositae).

360. Kleiman, R., M. H. Rawls and F. R. Earle

1972 *Cis*-5-monoenoic fatty acids in some Chenopodiaceae seed oils. *Lipids* 7(7):494-496.

361. Kleiman, R., R. W. Miller, F. R. Earle and I. A. Wolff

1966 Optically active aceto-triglycerides of oil from *Euonymus verrucosus* seed. *Lipids* 1(4):286-287.

362. —.

1967 (*S*)-1, 2-Diacyl-3-acetins: optically active triglycerides from *Euonymus verrucosus* seed oil. *Lipids* 2(6):473-478.

363. Kneebone, W. R. and V. G. Heller

1956 Leaf and crude protein percentages among strains of some forage grasses. Okla. Agr. Exp. Sta. *Tech. Bulletin*, T65, 23 pp.

364. Knievel, D. P. and D. Smith

1970 Yields and chemical composition of timothy (*Phleum pratense* L.) plants derived from summer and winter tillers. *Crop. Science* 10:270-273.

365. Knight, H. G., F. E. Hepner and A. Nelson

1911 Wyoming forage plants and their chemical composition-studies No. 4, Wyo. Agr. Exp. Sta. *Bulletin,* 87, 152 pp.

366. Knowles, R. E., K. W. Taylor, G. O. Kohler and L. A. Goldblatt

1964 Hydroxy-unsaturated oils and meal from *Dimorphotheca* and *Lesquerella* seed. *J. Agr. Food Chem.* 12:390-392.

367. Kovacevic, J., J. Cizek and V. Kurjakovic

1963 [*Rubus ulmifolius* Schott, *Portulaca oleracea* L. and *Agave americana* L. as fodder plant for pigs.] *Veterinaria Sarajevo* 12:369-372. Serbian: English Summary.

Nutr. Abstr., 34:3844.

Proximate analysis: Species: *Rubus* berries, *Portulaca* leaves and stems, *Agave*-peeled and chopped leaves.

368. —.

1967 [*Heracleum sphondylium* L. and *Lappa officinalis* All. as fodder plants]. *Veterinaria Sarajevo* 16:551-554. Serbo-Croat: English Summary.

Nutr. Abstr., 38:4506.

Crude fiber and protein reported.

Species: *Portulaca oleracea* parts above ground, *Agave americana* mesophil, 2 species of Rubus stems, leaves and fruits, and *Asphodelus albus* leaves.

369. Kozlowski, T. T.

    1958   Tree Physiology Bibliography. U.S.D.A., Washington, D.C.

370. Kramer, P. J. and T. T. Kozlowski

    1960   Physiology of Trees. McGraw-Hill, Inc. New York.

371. Krampitz, G., W. Haas and H. Hardebeck

    1970   [Lysine-rich proteins in leaves and seeds of *Atriplex hortensis*]. *Ztsohr. Tierphysiol. Tierernahrung Fattermittelk.* 27:1-9. German: English Summary.

    Nutr. Abstr., 41:4967.

372. Kretchmer, A. E., Jr., V. A. Lazar and K. C. Beeson

    1954   A preliminary survey of the cobalt contents of South Florida forages. *Soil Sci. Soc. Florida, Proc.* XIV:53-57.

373. Krewson, C. F., J. S. Ard and R. W. Riemenschneider

    1962   *Vernonia anthelmintica* (L.) Willd. Trivernolin, 1, 3-civernolin and vernolic (epoxyoleic) acid from the seed oil. *J. Amer. Oil. Chemists Soc.* 41:422-426.

374. Krochmal, A., et al.

    1972   Lobeline content of four Appalachian lobelias. *Lloydia* 35:303-304.

375. Krochmal, A., S. Paur and P. Duisberg

    1954   Useful native plants in the American southwestern deserts. *Econ. Bot.* 8(1):3-20.

376. Krueger, Kenneth W.

> 1967 Nitrogen, phosphorous and carbohydrate in expanding and year-old Douglas-fir shoots. *For. Sci.* 13(4):352-356.
>
> Mg/gm dry weight by month (March-June) for N, P, and carbohydrate; also given in mg/shoot total quantity.
>
> Species: *Pseudotsuga menziesii* (Mirb.) Franco.

377. Krueger, Kenneth W. and J. M. Trappe

> 1967 Food reserves and seasonal growth of Douglas-fir seedlings. *For. Sci.* 13(2):192-202.
>
> Tops and roots sugars, starch, crude fat, protein mg/gm dry weight; graphs of biweekly shoot elongation, stem diameter and root activity.
>
> Species: *Pseudotsuga menziesii* (Mirb.) Franco.

378. Kubota, J.

> 1964 Cobalt content of New England soils in relation to cobalt levels in forages for ruminant animals. *Soil Sci. Soc. Amer. Proc.* 28:246-251.
>
> The relationships of Co contents in red clover and alsike clover, and in red clover and alfalfa sampled from widely different soils of New England (according to drainage and soil morphology).

379. Kubota, J., E. R. Lemon and W. H. Allaway

> 1963 The effect of soil moisture content upon the uptake of Mo, Cu, and Co by alsike clover. *Soil Sci. Soc Amer. Proc.* 27:679-683.

380. Kubota, J., S. Rieger and V. A. Lazar

1970   Mineral composition of herbage browsed by moose in Alaska. *J. Wildl. Mgmt.* 34(3):565-569.

N, P, S, K, Ca, Co, Cu, Zn, Mn, Mo, Se (browse plants as a group), Cd is selected samples. Seasonal change of N in leaves and twigs reported.

Species: Leaves of *Salix* spp., *Populus tremuloides, Betula papyrifera* var. *kenaica, B. glandulosa; Equisetum* spp.; Grasses: *Eriophorum angustifolium* and *Calamagrostis canadensis;* Forbs: *Epilobium angustifolium* and *Lupinus* sp. Twigs of *Salix* spp., *Populus tremuloides, Betula papyrifera* ver. *kenaica, B. glandulosa.*

381. Kubota, J., V. A. Lazar and K. C. Beeson

1960   The study of cobalt status of soils in Arkansas and Louisiana using the black gum as the indicator plant. *Soil Sci. Soc. Amer. Proc.* 24:527-528.

Wide range of concentration in leaves (1-900 ppm) using technique of foliar analysis.

382. Kupchan, S. M., et al.

1973   New alkaloids and related artifacts from *Cyclea peltata. J. Org. Chem.* 38:1846-1852.

383. Kupchan, S. M., J. H. Zimmerman and A. Afonso

1961   The alkaloids and taxonomy of *Veratrum* and related genera. *Lloydia* 24(1):1-27.

384. Kuppers, J. R., L. L. Rusoff and D. M. Sneath

1948   Seasonal variations of carotene and other nutritionally

Kuppers, J. R., L. L. Rusoff and D. M. Sneath (cont.)

important constituents in the two pasture grasses Dallis and carpet. *J. Agr. Res.* 77:55-63.

Significant positive correlation exists between crude protein and crude carotene in Dallis and carpet grass over a 9 month growing season. Seasonal maxima of carotene, protein and Ca occured in spring in Dallis grass and in early summer in carpet grass.

385. Kurien, P. P.

1967 Distribution of protein, calcium and phosphorous between the husk and endosperm of rajgira seeds (*Amaranthus paniculatus*). *J. Nutr. Dietetics*, India 4:153-155.

Nutr. Abstr., 38:308.

L

386. Lachover, D. and Tadmor

1965 [Qualitative study of *Atriplex halimus* as a forage plant growing in semi-arid conditions in Israel. I. Seasonal changes in chlorides and essential minerals, and the presence of oxalates in different parts of the plant]. *Agronom. trop.* 20:309-322. French: English and Spanish Summaries.

Nutr. Abstr., 36:353.

Values given for NaCl, Na, K, Ca, Mg, Cl, S, P, and oxalate in leaves, stalks, fruit and branches.

100

387. Laessle, Albert M. and D. E. Frye, Jr.

1956   A food study of the Florida bobwhite. *J. Wildl. Mgmt.*
20(2):125-131.

Proximate and mineral (Ca, P) analysis of wax-myrtle
(*Myrica* spp.) and *Scleria muhlenbergii.*

388. Lajolo, F. M.

1967   [Waste products of sisal (*Agave sisalana*) as an animal
feed] . *Rev. Fac. Farm Bioquim.*, Sao Paulo 5:373-381.
Portuguese: English Summary.

Nutr. Abstr., 40:2537.

Analysis done after fiber removed; proximate components, Mn, K, Na, P, Fe and Cu (mg/100g fresh cut).

389. Lakshminarayana, S. and A. G. Mathew

1967   Leucoanthocyanidins of sapota fruit. *J. Food Sci.* 32(4):
451-452.

Sapodilla fruit.

390. Lambert, J. L., D. C. Clanton, I. A. Wolff and G. C. Mus-
takas

1970   Crambe meal protein and hulls in beef cattle rations. *J.
Anim. Sci.* 31(3):601-607.

391. Lambertsen, G., H. Myklestad and O. R. Braekkan

1962   Tocopherols in nuts. *J. Sci. Food Agric.* 13:617-620.

Nutr. Abstr., 33:2386.

Covers all of the common varieties of nuts.

392. Lawrence, T. and J. E. Troelsen

1964   An evaluation of 15 grass species as forage crops for southwestern Saskatchewan. *Canad. J. Plant Sci.* 44:301-310.

Nutr. Abstr., 35:1953.

Grasses evaluated for dry matter yield, protein content, *in vitro* digestibility of cellulose and winter hardiness.

Fifteen successive weekly cuttings and analyses made.

393. Leaf, A. L.

1964   Pure maple syrup: nutritive value. *Science* 143:963-964.

Nutr. Abstr., 34:5585.

Nitrogen and sugar content of both syrup and sap given. Syrup also analyzed for P, K, Ca and Mg (ppm).

Species: *Acer saccharum.*

394. Leaf, Albert L. and K. G. Watterson

1964   Chemical analysis of sugar maple sap and foliage as related to sap and sugar yields. *For. Sci.* 10(3):288-292.

Significant differences (.01 level) among groups of trees rated as very high, high, medium, low and very low producers of sap in ash concentrations and contents of foliage, and at the .05 level for N, K, Ca and P contents of foliage. Lower sap producers have higher concentrations in leaves. Also intra-seasonal analyses of both foliage and sap (ratio of sugar to N, P, K, Ca and Mg) reported.

395. Leaf, Albert L. and T. Keller

1956 Tentative techniques for determining the influence of soil on the growth of forest populations. *Proc. Amer. Soil Sci. Soc.* 20:1110-1112.

On fertile soil, N and P concentrations in red pine foliage were 0.74 percent and 0.15 percent respectively.

396. Lech, W., K. Wichura and H. Losinska

1972 [Protein in foliage fallen from trees]. *Przemyst Fermentacyjnyi Rolny* 16(2):20-22. Polish: Russian and English Summary.

Nutr. Abstr., 42:8021.

Maple leaves analyzed. Amino acids and sugar components reported.

397. Lessard, J. R., M. Hidiroglou, R. B. Carson and P. Dermine

1968 Intra-seasonal variations in the selenium content of various forage crops at Kapuskasing, Ontario. *Canad. J. Plant. Sci.* 48:581-585.

Nutr. Abstr., 39:4622.

Se content of 5 grasses of *Lotus corniculatus* L. (trefoil), at each of two harvests made 7 weeks apart, June-September. Se content of orchard grass, timothy and birdsfoot trefoil plotted.

398. Leung, Woot-Tsuen Wu and M. Flores

1961 *Food Composition Table for Use in Latin America*, INCAP-ICNND, National Institutes of Health, Bethesda, Maryland.

399. Levin, Donald A.

1974 The oil content of seeds: an ecological perspective. *Amer. Naturalist* 108(960):193-206.

Seed oil content (mean oil content percentage dry weight) and mean seed weight of approx. 100 plant families, representing more than 1300 species. The species chosen are representatives of a world wide flora.

400. Lewis, R. D. and R. L. Lang

1957 Effect of nitrogen on yield of forage of eight grasses grown in high altitude meadows of Wyoming. *Agron. J.* 49:332-335.

Percent crude protein (dry wt. basis) plotted against nitrogen (in lbs. per acre annually). Percent P and percent Ca plotted similarly.

Species: Common brome, Lincoln brome, Manchar brome, intermediate wheat grass, meadow foxtail, orchard grass, reed canary grass and timothy hay.

401. Leyton, L.

1956 The relationship between the growth and mineral composition of the foliage of Japanese larch (*Larix leptolepis,* Murr.). *Plant and Soil* 7:167-177.

There exists a significant relationship between the amount of nitrogen and phosphorous in the foliage and height growth.

402. Leyton, L. and K. A. Armson

1955 Mineral composition of the foliage in relation to growth of Scots pine. *Forest Sci.* 1:210-218.

Leyton, L. and K. A. Armson (cont.)

> N, P, K, Ca and other (combined) ash constituents. Multiple regression equations indicate N and P content correlate strongly with tree growth (for terminal foliage). Multiple correlation coefficient = 0.972.

403. Lichtenstein, E. P., D. G. Morgan and C. H. Mueller

> 1964   Naturally occurring insecticides in cruciferous crops. *J. Agric. Food Chem.* 12:158-161.

> Nutr. Abstr., 34:5570.

404. Lichtenstein, E. P. and J. E. Casida

> 1963   Myristicin, an insecticide and synergist occuring naturally in the edible parts of parsnips. *J. Agric. Food Chem.* 11: 410-415.

> Nutr. Abstr., 34:2131.

> Five-allyl-1-methoxy-2,3-methylenedioxybenzene (approximate concentration 200 ppm).

405. Lima, I. H., T. Richardson and M. A. Stahmann

> 1965   Fatty acids in some leaf protein concentrates. *J. Agric. Food Chem.* 13:143-145.

> Nutr. Abstr., 35:5525.

> Species: Chenopodium, red clover, rye grass and various cultigens analyzed.

406. Lindahl, I., R. E. Davis and W. O. Shepard

> 1949   The application of the total available carbohydrate meth-

Lindahl, I., R. E. Davis and W. O. Shepard (cont.)

od to the study of carbohydrate reserves of switch cane
(*Arundinaria tecta*). *Plant Physiol.* 24(2):285-294.

407. Lingaiah, Sushela

1952   The nutritional evaluation of certain nut proteins (walnuts
and pecans). Mich. State College Ph.D. Thesis.

408. Litchfield, C.

1970   Taxonomic patterns in the fat content, fatty acid composition and triglyceride composition of Palmae seeds.
Chem. Phys. Lipids 4:96-103.

Nutr. Abstr., 40:7116.

There is a direct correlation between composition and the
botanical sub-families within the Palmae.

409. Litchfield, J. H., V. G. Vely and R. C. Overbeck

1963   Nutrient content of morel mushroom mycelium; amino
acid composition of the protein. *J. Food Sci.* 28:741-
743.

Nutr. Abstr., 34:3878.

410. Lopez, H., J. M. Navia, D. Clement and R. S. Harris

1963   Nutrient composition of Cuban foods. 3. Foods of vegetable origin. *J. Food Sci.* 28:600-610.

Nutr. Abstr., 34:2112.

Proximate content of 59 species and varieties.

411. Low, Jessop B. and F. C. Bellrose, Jr.

1944 The seed and vegetative yield of waterfowl food plants in the Illinois River Valley. *J. Wildl. Mgmt.* 8(1):7-22.

Seed yield cc./m^2: foliage production of 6 submerged species.

Species: *Echinocloa crus-galli, E. frumentacea, E. walteri, Cephalanthus occidentalis, Zizania aquatica, Pontederia cordata, Sparganium eurycarpum, Potamogeton americanus, P. pectinatus, Polygonum pennsylvanicum, P. hydropiperoides, P. punctatum, Cyperus esculentus, C. strigosus, C. erythrorhizos, Acnida tuberculata, Leersia oryzoides, Lophotocarpus calycinus, Sagittaria latifolia, Eragrostis hypnoides, E. pectinacea, Scirpus validus, S. americanus, S. acutus, S. fluviatilis, Nelumbo lutea, Polygonum muhlenbergii, Potamogeton pusillus, Ceratophyllum demersum.*

412. Lowry, G. L. and P. M. Avard

1965 Nutrient content of black spruce needles. I. Variations due to crown position and needle age. *Woodland Research Index*, Pulp and Paper Research Inst., Canada, No. 171, 21 pp.

413. Lund, A. P. and W. M. Sandstrom

1943 The proteins of various tree seeds. *J. Agr. Res.* 66(9): 349.

Proximate analysis of various oaks, ironwood and elm. Data reported for protein (albumin, globulin and glutelin fractions) and nitrogen distribution as well.

414. Lunt, H. A.

1935 Effect of weathering upon dry matter and composition of

Lunt, H. A. (cont.)

hardwood leaves. *J. For.* 33:607-609.

Comparison of fresh and weathered leaves for percent Ash, Ca, K, P, and N in 6 species of trees. Beech, red maple, sugar maple, hickory, white oak and dogwood.

M

415. Maarse, Henry and R. E. Kepner

1970　Changes in composition of volatile terpenes in Douglas-fir needles during maturation. *J. Agric. Food Chem.* 18: 1095-1101.

No variation in cyclic oxygenated monoterpenes. Increase with age of acyclic oxygenated monoterpenes. Discussion of palatability and effects of fertilization with urea vs. gypsum on composition.

416. McCall, Ralph

1939　Seasonal variation in the composition of blue bunch fescue. *J. Agr. Res.* 58:603-616.

Proximate contents, Ca and P.

Species:　*Festuca idahoensis* Elmer.

417. McCall, Ralph, R. T. Clark and A. R. Patton

1943　The apparent digestibility and nutritive value of several native and introduced grasses. Mont. Agr. Exp. Sta. *Bulletin,* 418, 30 pp.

418. McCarty, E. C.

    1938   The relationship of growth to the varying carbohydrate content in mountain brome. U.S. Dept. Agr. *Tech. Bulletin,* 598, 27 pp.

419. McCarty, E. C. and R. Price

    1942   Growth and carbohydrate content of important mountain forage plants in central Utah as affected by clipping and grazing. U.S. Dept. Agr. *Tech. Bulletin,* 818, 51 pp.

           Species: Two perennial grasses: Mountain brome and slender wheatgrass; 2 broadleaf plants: sticky geranium and niggerhead.

420. McCarty, Edward C.

    1938   Seasonal march of the carbohydrates in *Elymus ambiguus* and *Muhlenbergia gracilis* and their relation under moderate grazing use. *Plant Phys.* 10:727-738.

421. McClean, A. and E. W. Tisdale

    1960   Chemical composition of native forage plants in British Columbia in relation to grazing practice. *Canadian J. Plant Sci.* 40:405-423.

           Crude protein, crude fiber, total ash, Ca, P and Ca/P ratio reported for 4 stages of growth (leaf, flower, seed and weathered).

           Species: Nine grasses, and 8 species of secondary grazing plants.

422. McComb, Elizabeth A. and V. V. Rendig

    1970   Some nonfermentable free carbohydrates in the leaves of

McComb, Elizabeth A. and V. V. Rendig (cont.)

canary grass (*Phalaris tuberosa*). *J. Agr. Food Chem.* 18:1092-1094.

Nutr. Abstr., 41:4975.

Comparison made of chromatographic data for various nonfermentable sugars and some authentic carbohydrates.

423. McConnell, B. R., and G. A. Garrison

1966   Seasonal variations of available carbohydrates in bitterbrush. *J. Wildl. Mgmt.* 30(1):168-172.

Nutr. Abstr., 36:5886.

All sugars, starch and dextrin which are mobilizable and available within the plant are reported upon (i.e. tops and roots are analyzed for available carbohydrates).

Species: *Purshia tridentata.*

424. McCreary, O. C.

1927   Wyoming forage plants and their chemical composition. Studies No. 8, Wyo. Exp. Sta. *Bulletin,* 157:91-105.

425. —.

1939   Phosphorous in Wyoming pasture, hay, and other foods. Wyo. Agr. Exp. Sta. *Bulletin,* 233, 20 pp.

426. McEwen, Lowell C.

1962   Leaf longevity and crude protein content for roughleaf rice grass in the Black Hills. *J. Range Mgmt.* 15(2):106-107.

McEwen, Lowell C. (cont.)

Graphs of average length of leaf through time, longevity of leaves (0-25 months) and crude protein content of leaves at various stages of maturity.

427. McEwen, Lowell C. and D. R. Dietz

1965   Shade effects on chemical composition of herbage in the Black Hills. *J. Range Mgmt.* 18(4):184-190.

Proximate analyses over 6 month period of *Poa pratensis* from open meadow and pine shaded sites.

428. McGee, Charles E.

1963   A nutritional study of slash pine seedlings grown in sand culture. *For. Sci.* 9(4):461-469.

Thirty rates of N, P and K supplies over 4 month period. Report of analysis for each formulation of the N, P and K content of shoots and roots. N affects fresh yield wt.; K affects dry wt. and seedling elongation. Percent N, P and K in shoot and root tissue increased with each increment of nutrient supply. N tends to increase at the greatest rate in shoots, P and K in roots.

429. McHargue, J. S. and W. R. Roy

1932   Mineral and nitrogen content of the leaves of some forest trees at different times in the growing seasons. *Botan. Gaz.* 94:381-393.

Analysis of leaves of 23 species collected at three intervals during the growing season. Data reported includes crude ash, insoluble residue (SiO_2), Cu, Fe, Mn, Zn, Ca, Mg, P, K, Na, S, N, protein, ether extract, and crude fiber as percentages of moisture-free material.

430. McIlvanie, S. K.

1942   Carbohydrate and nitrogen trends in blue bunch wheat grass, *Agropyron spicatum,* with special reference to grazing influences. *Plant Physiol.* 17:540-547.

431. McKell, Cyrus M., R. Derwyn Whalley and V. Brown

1966   Yield, survival, and carbohydrate reserve of harding grass in relation to herbage removal. *J. Range Mgmt.* 19(2): 86-89.

Report of carbohydrate values as mean of six plants under various clipping schedules (on percent dry matter basis).

432. Mackie, W. W.

1903   The value of oak leaves for forage. Univ. of Calif. Agr. Exp. Sta. *Bulletin,* 150, 21 pp.

433. McNair, J. B.

1930   The taxonomic and climatic distribution of oil and starch in seeds in relation to the physical and chemical properties of both substances. *Am. J. Bot.* 17(7):662-668.

Two-hundred and sixteen families rated. Taxonomic and climatic distribution of starch and oil in seeds is discussed.

434. Madgwick, H. A. I.

1964   Variations in the composition of red pine (*Pinus resinosa* Ait.) leaves: a comparison of well-grown and poorly-grown trees. *Forestry* 37(1):87-94.

Report of changes in needle nutrient distribution with position in crown (P, K, N, Ca, Mg and Ash) for well-grown and poorly-grown trees. Also, data regarding

112

Madgwick, H. A. I. (cont.)

changes in concentration with ages of needles with respect to K, P, Ca, Mg, N and ash for poorly-grown and well-grown trees.

435. Marvin, J. W., M. Morselli and F. M. Laing

1967   A correlation between sugar concentration and volume yields in sugar maple—an 18-year study. *For. Sci.* 13(4): 346-351.

Acer saccharum data; percent sugar per ltr. and total sap volume from 27 trees over 14 years. Also; percent sugar concentration from single tap holes (1 per tree).

436. Masada, Y., K. Hashimoto, T. Inoue and M. Suzuki

1971   Analysis of the pungent principles of *Capsicum annuum* by combined gas chromatography-mass spectrometry. *J. Food Sci.* 36(6):858-860.

Nutr. Abstr., 42:5347.

437. May, J. T., H. H. Johnson and A. R. Gilmore

1962   Chemical composition of southern pine seedlings. *Ga. For. Res. Comm. Res. Paper,* 10, 11 pp.

P, K, Ca, Mg, Na, N (% dry matter) in needles, stems, roots and entire plant.

Species: *Pinus taeda* L., *P. elliotii* var. *elliottii, P. palustris* Mill.

438. Maynard, L. A.

1937   Interpretations of variations in plant composition in rela-

113

Maynard, L. A. (cont.)

tion to feeding value. *J. Amer. Soc. Agron.* 29(3):504-
511.

439. Melhus, Irving E., F. Aguirre and N. S. Scrimshaw

1953 Observations on the nutritive value of teosinte. *Science*
117:34-35.

Hulled teosinte from Jutiapa, Guatemala and a commercial variety from Florida, U.S.A., compared to a U.S. hybrid corn and Tiquisate Golden Yellow, a flint from Anti-
gua, Guatemala.

Analyzed for fat, N, Methionine, Lysine, Tryptophane
and Niacin.

Conclusion: N value of Teosinte higher than corn; methionine value of teosinte 2x that of corn.

440. Messer, Ellen

1972 Patterns of "wild" plant consumption in Oaxaca, Mexico.
Ecology of Food and Nutrition, Vol. I, pp. 325-332.

Descriptive article—recipes for *Amaranthus hybridus,
Anoda cristata, Chenopodium ambrosioides, Chenopodium* sp., *Crotolaria pumila, Galinsoga parviflora, Lippia
alba, Malva parviflora, Opuntia* sp., *Porophyllum tage-
loides, Portulaca oleracea* and *Tridax coronopifolia.*

441. Miaki, T.

1967 [Studies on chemical composition and feeding value in
forage crops: 9. An influence of level of nitrogen fertilization, stage of maturity and growth phase on chemical
composition and feeding value of Bahia grass. 10. An influence of nitrogen fertilization and stage of maturity on

Miaki, T. (cont.)

chemical composition and feeding value of teosinte forage. (*Euchlaena mexicana* Schrad.).] Note: for "10" see Nutr. Abstr. 38:2376.

Jap. J. Zootech. Sci. 38:187-193, 252-256. Japanese: English summary and tables.

442. Midgley, R. A.

1937 Modification of chemical composition of pasture plants by soils. *J. Amer. Soc. Agron.* 29:498-503.

443. Miettinen, J. K. and A. I. Virtanen

1952 The free amino acids in the leaves, roots and root nodules of the alder (*Alnus*). *Physiol. Plant.* 5:540-557.

444. Mikolajczak, K. L. and C. R. Smith, Jr.

1967 Pentacyclic triterpenes of *Jurinea anatolica* Boiss. and *Jurinea consanguinea* DC. fruit. *Lipids* 2(2):127-132.

445. —.

1967 Optically active trihydroxy acids of *Chamaepeuce* seed oils. *Lipids* 2(3):261-265.

446. —.

1968 Penta-acid triglycerides of *Chamaepeuce afra* seed oil. *Biochem. Biophys. Acta* 152(2):244-254.

447. Mikolajczak, K. L. and C. R. Smith, Jr.

1971   Cyanolipids of Kusum (*Schleichera trijuga*) seed oil. *Lipids* 6(5):349-350.

448. Mikolajczak, K. L., C. R. Smith, Jr. and I. A. Wolff

1963   Three new oilseeds rich in *Cis*-11-Eicosenoic acid. *J. Am. Oil Chemists' Soc.* 40(7):294-295.

1) *Marshallia caespitosa* Nutt. (Compositae) seed oil contains 44% *Cis*-11-Eicosenoic acid (C_{20}-monoenoic acid).

2) *Alyssum maritimum* (L.) Lam. (Cruciferae) seed oil contains 42% *Cis*-11-Eicosenoic acid.

3) *Selenia grandis* Martin (Cruciferae) seed oil contains 58% *Cis*-11-Eicosenoic acid.

Bibliography includes references to other genera containing this particular fatty acid.

449. —.

1965   Dihydroxy fatty acids in *Cardamine impatiens* seed oil. *J. Am. Oil Chemists' Soc.* 42(11):939-941.

450. —.

1968   Glyceride structure of *Cardamine impatiens* L. seed oil. *Lipids* 3(3):215-220.

451. —.

1970   Phenolic and sugar components of Armavirec variety sunflower (*Hellianthus annuus*) seed meal. *J. Agr. Food Chem.* 18(1):27-32.

452. Mikolajczak, K. L., C. R. Smith, Jr. and L. W. Tjarks

1970 Cyanolipids of *Stocksia brahuica* Benth. seed oil. *Biochim. Biophys. Acta.* 210(2):305-314.

453. —.

1970 Cyanolipids of *Koelreuteria paniculata* Laxm. seed oil. *Lipids* 5(8):672-677.

Member of the Sapindaceae.

454. —.

1970 Cyanolipids of *Cardiospermum halicacabum* L. and other sapindaceous seed oils. *Lipids* 5(10):812-817.

455. Mikolajczak, K. L., D. S. Seigler, C. R. Smith, Jr., I. A. Wolff and R. B. Bates

1969 A cyanogenetic lipid from *Cordia verbenacea* DC seed oil. *Lipids* 4(6):617-619.

456. Mikolajczak, K. L., F. R. Earle and I. A. Wolff

1962 Search for new industrial oils VI. Seed oils of the genus *Lesquerella*. *J. Am. Oil Chemists' Soc.* 39(2):78-80.

457. —.

1963 The acetylenic acid in *Comandra pallida* and *Osyris alba* seed oils. *J. Am. Oil Chemists' Soc.* 40(8):342-343.

458. Mikolajczak, K. L., M. F. Rogers, C. R. Smith, Jr. and I. A. Wolff

    1967   An octadecatrienoic acid from *Lamium purpureum* L. seed oil containing 5, 6-allenic and *Trans*-16-olefinic unsaturation. *Biochem. J.* 105(3):1245-1249.

459. Mikolajczak, K. L., R. M. Freidinger, C. R. Smith, Jr. and I. A. Wolff

    1968   Oxygenated fatty acids of oil from sunflower seeds after prolonged storage. *Lipids* 3(6):489-494.

460. Mikolajczak, K. L., T. K. Miwa, F. R. Earle, I. A. Wolff and Q. Jones

    1961   Search for new industrial oils V. Oils of Cruciferae. *J. Am. Oil Chemists' Soc.* 38(12):678-681.

461. Milford, R.

    1960   Nutritional values of 17 subtropical grasses. *Austral. J. Agr. Res.* 11(2):138-149.

462. Miller, D. F.

    1958   Composition of cereal grain and forages. National Research Council, Washington, D.C., Pub. 585.

463. Miller, E. C.

    1938   *Plant Physiology.* McGraw-Hill Book Co., New York. Minerals (minor elements) in plants. Of historical value.

464. Miller, R. W., C. H. Van Etten and I. A. Wolff

  1962 Amino acid composition of *Lesquerella* seed meals. *J. Am. Oil Chemists' Soc.* 39(2):115-117.

465. Miller, R. W., F. R. Earle, I. A. Wolff and Q. Jones

  1964 Search for new industrial oils. IX. *Cuphea,* a versatile source of fatty acids. *J. Am. Oil Chemists' Soc.* 41(4): 279-280.

466. Miller, R. W., M. E. Daxenbichler, F. R. Earle and H. S. Gentry

  1964 Search for new industrial oils. VIII. The genus *Limnanthes. J. Am. Oil Chemists' Soc.* 41(3):167-169.

467. Miller, Roger Wayne, C. H. Van Etten, C. McGrew, I. A. Wolff and Q. Jones

  1962 Amino acid composition of seed meals from forty-one species of Cruciferae. *J. Agr.* and *Food Chem.* 10:426-430.

468. Miller, Roger Wayne, F. R. Earle, I. A. Wolff and A. S. Barclay

  1968 Search for new seed oils. XV. Oils of Boraginaceae. *Lipids* 3(1):43-45.

469. Miller, Roger Wayne, F. R. Earle, I. A. Wolff and Q. Jones

  1965 Search for new industrial oils. XIII. Oils from 102 species of Cruciferae. *J. Am. Oil Chemists' Soc.* 42(10:817-821.

470. Miller, W. J., W. E. Adams, R. Nussbaumer, R. A. McCreery and H. F. Perkins

1964 Zinc content of coastal bermuda grass as influenced by frequency and season of harvest, location and level of N and lime. *Agron. J.* 56:198-201.

Species: *Cynodon dactylon* (L.) Pers.

471. Milner, R. T., J. E. Hubbard and M. B. Wiele

1945 Sunflower and Safflower seeds and oils. *Oil and Soap* 22(11):304-307.

472. Miltimore, J. E. and J. L. Mason

1971 Copper to molybdenum ratio and molybdenum and copper concentrations in ruminant feeds. *Canad. J. Anim. Sci.* 51(1):193-200.

Nutr. Abstr., 42:316.

Grass and sedge hays analyzed; also: legume hay, legume-grass hay, oat forage, maize silage, and grains of Br. Columbia.

473. Misra, P. S., M. Pal, C. R. Mitra and T. N. Khoshoo

1971 Chemurgic studies on some diploid and tetraploid grain amaranths. *Proceedings of the Indian Acad. Sci.* (1971) 74B(3):155-160.

Nutr. Abstr., 42:2952.

Five species of *Amaranthus* treated with colchicine. Proteine, fat, reducing and non-reducing sugars, amino acids.

474. Mitchell, H. L.

1936   Trends in the nitrogen, phosphorous, potassium and calcium content of the leaves of some forest trees during growing season. *Black Rock Forest Papers* 1(6):30-44.

N, P, K, Ca, H_2O, dry wt. increase of leaves during growing season analyzed.

Leaves from the same portion of each tree analyzed (nutrients vary with leaf-position).

Species: New York trees—data compared to trees from Minnesota. *Quercus alba* L., *Q. montana* Wild, *Q. borealis* Michx., *Hicoria ovata* (Mill.) Britton, *Acer saccharum* Marsh, *A. rubrum, Picea abies L.*

475. Mitchell, H. L. and R. F. Finn

1935   The relative feeding power of oaks and maples for soil phosphorous. *Black Rock Forest Papers* 1(2):6-9.

Plot of percentage P in leaves of trees grown on soils with varying rates of rock phosphate fertilizer indicates same qualitative relationship (same positive slope of percentage/conc. P) for these two genera, but a quantitative difference exists for actual quantity of phosphate taken up by each genera.

Species: *Quercus borealis* Michx., *Acer rubrum* L.

476. Monarca, C. J. and E. V. Lynn

1937   Acorns of *Quercus rubra*. *J. of Amer. Pharmaceutical Assn.* 26(6):493-495, Easton, Pennsylvania.

477. Montgomery, C. R., H. D. Ellzey, M. Allen and L. L. Rusoff

1972   Effect of age and seasons on the quality of bahia grass.

Montgomery, C. R., H. D. Ellzey, M. Allen and L. L. Rusoff
(cont.)

La. Agr. 15(3):8-9, 11.

Nutr. Abstr., 42:8028.

478. Mooney, H. A. and W. D. Billings

1960   The annual carbohydrate cycle of alpine plants as related
        to growth. *Amer. J. Bot.* 47(7):594-598.

        Saxifraga rhomboidea, Polygonum bistortoides and *Geum
        turbinatum,* plotted for 1 year tot. CHO, tot. sugar, and
        starch for leaves, rhizomes and/or roots. Also given are
        root CHO contents (percent on basis of dry alcohol-in-
        soluble residue wt.) for *Pulsatilla ludoviciana, Lewisia
        pygmea, Carex elynoides, Luzula spicata.*

479. Morrison, Frank B.

1956   *Feeds and Feeding.* 22nd Edit., Ithaca, N.Y., Morrison
        Publ. Co., 1165 pp.

        Appendix containing proximate contents of many feeds
        and feeding stuffs.

480. Morton, Julia F.

1962   Spanish needles (*Bidens pilosa* L.) as a wild food resource.
        Econ. Bot. 16:173-179.

        Proximate contents.

481. Mowat, D. N., R. S. Fulkerson, W. E. Tossell and J. E.
     Winch

1965   The *in vitro* digestibility and protein content of leaf and

122

Mowat, D. N., R. S. Fulkerson, W. E. Tossell and J. E. Winch (cont.)

stem portions of forages. *Canad. J. of Plant Sci.* 45:321-331.

Nutr. Abstr., 36:2250.

Timothy, cocksfoot, bromegrass and lucerne. Crude protein contents of leaf and stem portions averaged over 3 years.

482. Mulay, M. S.

1931 Seasonal changes in total, soluble, soluble-protein, and insoluble nitrogen in current year's shoots of Barlett pear. *Plant Physiol.* 6:519-529.

483. Munsell, H. E., L. O. Williams, L. P. Guild, C. B. Troescher, G. Nightgale and R. S. Harris

1949 Composition of food plants of Central America. I. *Food Research* 14:144-164.

1950a Composition of food plants of Central America. II. *Food Research* 15:16-33.

1950b Composition of food plants of Central America. III. *Food Research* 15:34-52.

484. Murphy, Dean A. and J. H. Ehrenreich

1965 Fruit-producing trees and shrubs in Missouri's Ozark Forests. *J. Wildl. Mgmt.* 29(3):497-503.

Relation of overstory crown cover and position on slope to species abundance and fruiting. Also gives table of plants per acre.

485. Muskat, E.

    1963 [Effect of temperature on the vitamin C content during
          growth of spinach dock, *Rumex patientia* L.] *Experientia*
          19:355-357. German: English Summary.

          Nutr. Abstr., 34:4022.

N

486. National Academy of Science—National Research Council

    1964 Joint United States-Canadian Tables of Feed Composi-
          tion. *Publ.* 1232, 167 pp.

487. Neal, W. M. and R. B. Becker

    1933 The composition of feedstuffs in relation to nutritional
          anemia in cattle. *J. Agr. Res.* 47:249-255.

          Proximate, Ca, Mg, P, and Fe contents of forage samples
          collected during the months of March-July. Mineral com-
          ponents are compared in samples taken in both healthy
          areas and salt-sick areas.

          Species: *Aristida stricta, Aristida* spp. (these have been
          sampled from both burned and unburned areas), alfalfa
          hay, beggarweed, lespedeza, Natal grass, soybeans, soy-
          bean silage, cornmeal, velvetbean seed, velvetbean feed
          meal, cottonseed meal (36 percent protein), and cotton-
          seed meal (43 percent protein).

488. Nelson, A. B., C. H. Herbel and H. M. Jackson

    1970 Chemical compositions of forage species grazed by cattle

124

Nelson, A. B., C. H. Herbel and H. M. Jackson (cont.)

on an arid New Mexico range. New Mexico State Univ.
Agr. Exp. Sta. *Bulletin*, 561, 33 pp.

489. Nelson, Maynard M., J. B. Moyle and A. T. Farnham

1966   Cobalt levels in foods and livers of pheasants. *J. Wildl.
Mgmt.* 30(2):423-425.

Co (ppm) in seeds of *Setaria* spp., *Ambrosia* spp., *Rosa*
spp. (rose hips), and corn.

490. Nesterov, V.

1964   [Nutritive values of some docks, species of the genus
Rumex, and their usefulness for feeding livestock],
Veterinaria, Sarajevo 13:125-128. Serbian: English
Summary.

Nutr. Abstr., 35:1947.

Proximate analysis.

Species: *Rumex crispus, R. acetosella, R. obtusifolius*
and *R. pulcher.*

491. Nestler, R. B., W. W. Bailey, A. C. Martin and H. E. McClure

1945   Value of wild feedstuffs for pen-reared bobwhite quail in
winter. *J. Wildl. Mgmt.* 9(2):115-120.

This article draws upon chemical analyses of King and
McClure (1944).

492. Nestler, Ralph B., J. V. Derby and J. B. DeWitt

1949   Vitamin A and carotene content of some wildlife foods.

125

Nestler, Ralph B., J. V. Derby and J. B. DeWitt (cont.)

J. Wildl. Mgmt. 13(3):271-274.

37 species of insects and other invertebrates and 26 species of seeds and fruits eaten by quail spectrophotometrically assayed for B-Carotene (I.U./gm.). *Chamaecrista, Bidens, Rumex, Polygonum, Ambrosia, Lespedeza* (5 sp.), *Glycine, Phaseolus, Symphoricarpos, Amorpha, Celastrus, Vitis, Euonymus, Solanum, Rosa, Rhus.*

Species and common names given in article as well.

493. Newlon, Chas. F., T. S. Baskett, R. P. Breitenbach and J. A. Stanford

1964 Sustaining values of emergency foods for bobwhites. *J. Wildl. Mgmt.* 28(3):532-542.

Proximate analysis, Ca and P for fruits and seeds of: *Lespedeza stipulacea, L. cuneata, Vigna sinensis, Setaria italica, Pennisetum glaucum, Zea mays, Sorghum vulgare, Rhus glabra, Rosa multiflora* (hips), and *Sassafras albidum.*

494. Nigam, S. N., J. I. Tu and W. B. McConnell

1969 Distribution of selenomethylselenocysteine and some other amino acids in species of *Astragalus,* with special reference to their distribution during the growth of *A. bisulcatus. Phytochemistry* 8:1161-1165.

Nutr. Abstr., 40:309.

495. Nunez, A.

1969 [Trace elements in Argentine soils and forages]. *Rev. Fac. Agronom. Vet.,* Buenos Aires, 1969, 17(3):7-14. Spanish: English Summary.

126

Nunez, A. (cont.)

Nutr. Abstr., 41:303.

Cu, Mo, Zn, Mn and Fe contents reported.

O

496. O'Dell, Boyd L., A. R. de Boland and S. R. Koirtyohann

1972 Distribution of phytate and nutritionally important elements among the morphological components of cereal grains. *J. Agr. Food Chem.* 20(3):718-721.

497. Oelberg, Kermit

1956 Factors affecting the nutritive value of range forage. *J. Range Mgmt.* 9(5):220-225.

Review.

498. Ogata, J. N., Y. Kawano, A. Bevenue and L. J. Casarett

1972 The ketoheptose content of some tropical fruits. *J. Agric. Food Chem.* 20(1):113-115.

Nutr. Abstr., 42:7991.

499. Oh, H. K., T. Sakai, M. B. Jones and W. M. Longhurst

1967 The effect of various essential oils isolated from Douglas-fir needles upon sheep and deer rumen microbial activity. *Appl. Microbiol.* 15:777-784.

127

500. Oh, John H., M. B. Jones, W. M. Longhurst and G. E. Connolly

1970   Deer browsing and rumen microbial fermentation of Douglas-fir as affected by fertilization and growth stage. *For. Sci.* 10(1):21-27.

Analysis covers three years following application of nitrogen fertilizer (also control plants without fertilizer). Also includes foliar analysis of old and new needles for crude protein (percentage dry basis), and manometric gas production in M moles/g.

Species: *Pseudotsuga menziesii.*

501. Olsson, G.

1960   Some relations between number of seeds per pod, seed size and oil content and the effect of selection for these characters in *Brassica* and *Sinapis*. *Hereditas* 46:29-70.

502. Orlandi, M. M. G., S. M. P. Furlanetto and M. De Vuono

1968   [Nutritional chemistry of *Diospyros kaki.* vars. *costata* and *mazelii*.]   *Rev. Fac. Farm. Bioquim,* Sao Paulo 6:45-52. Portuguese with English summary.

Nutr. Abstr., 40:2524.

Proximate analysis, Ca, Mg, Fe and P.

503. Orman, H. R. and G. M. Will

1960   The nutrient content of *Pinus radiata* trees. *New Zeal. J. Sci.* 3:510-522.

128

504. Orr, J. B.

1929   *Minerals in Pastures.* H. K. Lewis Co., London.

505. Ovington, J. D.

1956   The composition of tree leaves. *Forestry* 29:22-28.

Foliar analysis for Na, K, Ca, Mg, Fe, Mn, SiO_2, P, Ash, C and N (percent oven-dry weight).

Twelve genera (various species) of the British Isles, some having North American distribution.

506. —.

1957   The volatile matter, organic carbon, and nitrogen contents of tree species grown in close stands. *New Phytol.* 56(1): 1-11.

For sampled species volatile matter, carbon and nitrogen (Kg/ha.) as well as percentage dry weight at one meter above ground reported along with total weights of individual trees, and percentage oven dry weight.

507. —.

1959   The calcium and magnesium contents of tree species grown in close stands. *New Phytol.* 58(2):164-175.

Percentage ash, Ca and Mg at various heights in sample tree species, total weights per tree (canopy and bole) in grams and kg/ha.

508. —.

1959   Mineral content of plantations of *Pinus sylvestris* L. *Annals of Botany* 23:75-88.

129

Ovington, J. D. (cont.)

Na, K, Ca, Mg, P, and N reported for various portions of the trees (grouped by age) in both mg/100g and Kg/ha. Also analysis of nutrient uptake (kg/ha) and nutrient return (kg/ha).

Species: Scots pine.

509. Ovington, J. D. and H. A. I. Madgwick

1959   The sodium potassium and phosphorous contents of tree species grown in close stands. *New Phytol.* 57(3):273-284.

Na, K, P and percentage ash of tree samples taken at varied heights, total weights Na, K, P per sample tree (canopy and bole) for 3 forests and estimates made of Na, K and P, kg/ha.

P

510. Paech, K. and M. V. Tracey (editors)

1955   Modern methods of plant analyses. Vol. IV: 11, Springer Verlag, Berlin.

511. Park, Barry C.

1942   The yield and persistence of wildlife food plants. *J. Wildl. Mgmt.* 6(2):118-121.

Tabulation of 27 plants listing common, generic and specific names, number and size of plants, percentage of plants bearing, quantities produced, date of ripening,

Park, Barry C. (cont.)

maximum date of persistence, average date of ripening, years crop failed and variation for date and quantity (maximum for a 4-year period).

512. Parker, Johnson

1951 Moisture retention in leaves of conifers of the northern Rocky Mountains. *Bot. Gaz.* 113:210-216.

Table of moisture content of detached leaves as percentage dry wt. and percentage of leaves showing positive tetrazolium test after being hydrated (a rough measure of needle viability).

Species: Douglas-fir, ponderosa pine, arborvitae, white pine, grand fir, and Engelmann spruce.

513. —.

1956 Variations in copper, boron and manganese in leaves of *Pinus ponderosa. For. Sci.* 2(3):191-198.

ppm Cu, B and Mn per ash and per dry leaf reported.

514. —.

1957 Seasonal changes in some chemical and physical properties of living cells of *Pinus ponderosa* and their relation to freezing resistance. *Protoplasma* 48:147-163.

Analysis in February and May of fructose, glucose, sucrose and raffinose contents in *Pinus ponderosa* and in *P. monticola* leaves and bark.

515. —.

1958   Changes in sugars and nitrogenous compounds of tree barks from summer to winter. *Naturwiss.* 45:139.

Tables:

1) Percentage protein nitrogen in inner barks of species shown based on dry weight. 10 genera, 12 species August, October and December.

2) Sugar in tree barks (% x 10 of fresh wt.). Stachyose, raffinose, melezitose, sucrose, glucose and fructose. August and December, 1957. Nine genera.

516. —.

1959   Seasonal variations in sugars of conifers with some observations on cold resistance. *For. Sci.* 5(1):56-63.

Report for various portions of the growing season of quantitative analyses for specific sugars (% of fresh weight x 10) in trunk, bark and leaves of *Pinus strobus, P. nigra, Picea abies, P. pungens, Thuja plicata* and *Tsuga canadensis.* Data are also given for the roots and branches (wood and bark) of *Pinus strobus.* Sugars analyzed for: stachyose, raffinose, sucrose, glucose and fructose. Qualitative test for presence of starch in various portions of *P. strobus* at various times during the growing season.

517. Patton, A. R.

1943   Seasonal changes in the lignin and cellulose content of some Montana grasses. *J. Animal Sci.* 2:59.

Percentage lignin and cellulose given at various stages of maturity for: *Agropyron cristatum* (L.) Gaertn, *A. pauciflorum* (Schwein) Hitch., *Bromus inermis* Leyss., *B. marginatus* Nees., *Arrhenatherum elatius* (L.) Mert. and Koch, *Bouteloua gracilis* (H.B.K.) Lag., *Elymus junceus* Fisch., *Festuca elatior* (L.) (var. arundinacea).

518. Patton, A. R. and L. Gieseker

1942   Seasonal changes in the lignin and cellulose content of some Montana grasses. *J. Animal Sci.* 1:22-26.

Percentage lignin and cellulose at various stages of maturity given for: *Agropyron cristatum* (L.) Gaertn., *A. pauciflorum* (Schwein) Hitch., *Bromus inermis* Leyss. *B. marginatus* Nees.

519. Paulsen, Harold A., Jr.

1969   Forage values on a mountain grassland—aspen range in Western Colorado. *J. Range Mgmt.* 22(2):102-107.

Crude protein, P and Ca of 9 major forage species calculated for vegetative stage, flowering stage, seed ripening and dispersal stage and regrowth-dormancy stage.

520. Pechnik, E. and L. R. Guimaraes

1961   [I Content of foods in common use in Brazil. 3. Leafy vegetables.] *Arq. brasil. Nutricao* 17(2):11-16. Portuguese: English and French Summaries.

Nutr. Abstr., 34:254.

521. —.

1962   [Some plants with high vitamin A potency.] *Univ. Brazil Inst. Nutricao Trab. Pesq.* 6:65-77. Portuguese: English and French Summaries.

Nutr. Abstr., 33:5944.

522. —.

1963   [I Content of foods eaten in Brazil. 4. Vegetables and

Pechnik, E. and L. R. Guimaraes (cont.)

> tubers.] *Arq. brasil. Nutricao* 19:11-16.

> Nutr. Abstr., 35:3629.

> Species: *Sonchus oleraceus* L., etc.

523. Pendergast, B. A.

> 1969 Nutrition of spruce grouse of the Swan Hills, Alberta. M.S. Thesis. Univ. of Alberta, 73 pp.

> See: Gurchinoff and Robinson, 1972, *J. Wildl. Mgmt.* 36(1):80.

524. Percival, G. P., D. Josselyn and K. C. Beeson

> 1955 Factors affecting the micronutrient element content of some forages in New Hampshire. New Hampshire Agr. Exp. Sta. *Tech. Bulletin, 93.*

525. Petrides, George A., P. Parmalee and J. E. Wood

> 1953 Acorn production in east Texas. *J. Wildl. Mgmt.* 17(3): 380-382.

> Average number of acorns per 25 twigs tabulated for *Quercus stellata,* correlated with tree height diameter and crown size.

526. Pharis, R. P., R. L. Barnes and A. W. Naylor

> 1964 Effects of nitrogen level, calcium level and nitrogen source upon the growth and composition of *Pinus taeda* L. *Physiol. Plant.* 17:560-572.

527. Phillips, B. E. and C. R. Smith, Jr.

    1970   Glycerides of *Monnina emarginata* seed oil. *Biochim. Biophys. Acta* 218(1):71-82.

528. —.

    1972   Stereo specific analysis of triglycerides from *Monnina emarginata* seed oil. *Lipids* 7(3):215-217.

529. Phillips, B. E., C. R. Smith, Jr. and J. W. Hagemann

    1969   Glyceride structure of *Erlangea tomentosa* seed oil, a new source of vernolic acid. *Lipids* 4(6):473-477.

530. Phillips, B. E., C. R. Smith, Jr. and L. W. Tjarks

    1970   Fatty acids of *Monnina emarginata* seed oil. *Biochim. Biophys. Acta* 210(3):353-359.

531. Phillips, Bruce E., C. R. Smith, Jr. and L. W. Tjarks

    1970   (S)-13-hydroxy-*cis*-9, *trans*-11-octadecadienoic acid lactone, a 14-membered-ring compound from *Monnina emarginata* seed oil. *J. Org. Chem.* 35(6):1916-1919.

532. Phillips, Bruce E., C. R. Smith, Jr. and W. H. Tallent

    1971   Glycerides of *Limnanthes douglasii* seed oil. *Lipids* 6(2):93-99.

533. Phillips, M., B. L. Davis and H. D. Weihe

    1942   Composition of the roots and tops of timothy plants at successive stages of growth. *J. Agr. Res.* 64:533-546.

Phillips, M., B. L. Davis and H. D. Weihe (cont.)

> Composition of the timothy plant at successive stages of growth (ash, N, crude protein, methoxyl, alcohol-benzene extractives, hot water + 1% HC1 extractives, uronic acid, total furfural, pentosans, crude cellulose, furfural in crude cellulose, lignin, N in ash-free crude lignin, methoxyl in ash-free crude lignin and pectic substances).

> Species: *Phleum pratense* L.

534. Phillips, Max and B. Davis

> 1940 Hemicelluloses of alfalfa hay. *J. Agr. Res.* 60:775-780.

535. Phillips, T. G., D. G. Rotley and J. T. Sullivan

> 1960 Grass holocellulose, stepwise hydrolysis of grass holocellulose. *J. Agric. Food Chem.* 8(2):153.

> Type of grass not specified; determination of simple sugars, uronides, oligosaccharides, hemicelluloses.

536. Phillips, T. G. and T. O. Smith

> 1943 The composition of timothy. Pt. I. Young grass and hay. New Hampshire Agr. Exp. Sta. *Tech. Bulletin,* 81.

537. Philpot, C. W.

> 1970 Influence of mineral content on the pyrolysis of plant materials. *For. Sci.* 16(4):461-471.

> Ash, silica-free ash, P, Fe, K, Ca and Na content of various plants analyzed.

538. Pichard, P.

1898 Contribution a la recherche du manganese dans les miner-aux, les vegetaux, et les animaus. [Contribution to investigations on manganese in minerals, plants and animals]. *Compt. Rend. Acad. Sci. de Paris* 126(26):1882-1885.

Mostly of historical value.

539. Pickett, R. C.

1950 Variability of crude protein and carotene contents and their relations with other characters of brome-grass. (*Bromus inermis* Leyss.). *Agron. J.* 42(11):550-554.

540. Piez, K. A., F. Irreverre and H. L. Wolff

1956 The separation and determination of cyclic imino acids. *J. Biol. Chem.* 223:687.

Small amounts of hydroxyproline, pipecolic acid, proline and 5 hydroxy pipecolic acid are reported from the pericarp of Calavo brand dates.

541. Pirie, N. W.

1964 Novel protein sources for use as human food in wet, tropical regions. *Ier Congress International des Industries Alimentaires et Agricoles.* pp. 237-248.

542. —.

1966 The merits of food proteins from novel sources. *Sci. Prog. Oxf.* 54:401-412.

543. Plummer, B. E.

1953   Chemical composition of grasses and legumes in Maine. Maine Agr. Exp. Sta. *Bulletin,* 513.

544. Plut, D. L. and J. C. Werner

1967   [Effect of season and height of cutting on lignin content of Napier grass], *Bol. Indust. animal. Sao Paulo,* 1967, 24:175-184. Portuguese: English Summary.

Nutr. Abstr., 39:2412.

Season and height had no significant effect on the comparatively low lignin content of this grass.

Species: *Pennisetum purpureum* Schum.

545. Plut, D. L. and L. Melotti

1965/66   [Lignin content and other chemical components of jaragua and molasses grass.] *Bol. Indust. animal, Sao Paulo* 23:169-175. Portuguese: English Summary.

Nutr. Abstr., 38:2365.

Cut and analyzed (proximate) at 7 vegetative stages of growth.

Species: Two common pasture grasses of Sao Paulo State. *Hyparrhenia rufa* (Jaragua) and *Melinis minutiflora* (molasses grass).

546. Pop, C. E.

1967   [Chemical composition of mulberry leaves at different periods and their consumption availability.] *Sericicultura* 1967, 3(4):12-18.

Pop, C. E. (cont.)

From Abstr. Romanian Tech. Lit.

Nutr. Abstr., 39:2394.

547. Powell, Jeff

1970　Site factor relationships with volatile oils in big sagebrush. *J. Range Mgmt.* 23(1):42-46.

Volatile oil content varies on different sites from 3.5%-6.0% and is most highly correlated with sagebrush size and quantity of Mg and P in the "A" horizon (91% of variability). Big plants on favorable sites have the greatest amount of volatile oil. Volatile oils are not palatable to wildlife.

Species: *Artemisia tridentata.*

548. Powell, R. G. and C. R. Smith, Jr.

1965　A C_{17}-hydroxy-acid from the oil of *Acanthosyris spinescens. Chem. Ind.* (London) (11):470.

549. —.

1966　New acetylenic fatty acids from *Acanthosyris spinescens* seeds oil. *Biochem.* 5(2):625-631.

550. Powell, R. G., C. R. Smith, Jr., C. A. Glass and I. A. Wolff

1965　*Helichrysum* seed oil. II. Structure and chemistry of a new enynolic acid. *J. Org. Chem.* 30(2):610-615.

551. —.

    1966   New enynolic acids from *Acanthosyris:* Structures and chemistry. *J. Org. Chem.* 31(2):528-533.

552. Powell, R. G., C. R. Smith, Jr. and I. A. Wolff

    1965   *Helichrysum* seed oil. I. Separation and characterization of individual acids. *J. Am. Oil Chemists' Soc.* 42(3):165-169.

553. —.

    1967   *Cis*-5, *Cis*-9, *Cis*-12-octadecatrienoic and some unusual oxygenated acids in *Xeranthemum annuum* seed oil. *Lipids* 2(2):172-177.

554. Price, N. O. and J. T. Huber

    1964   Minor element content of forage plants from the Shenandoah Valley and Southwest Virginia. Virginia Agr. Exp. Sta. *Tech. Bulletin,* 177.

555. Price, N. O., W. N. Linkous and R. W. Engle

    1955   Minor element content of forage plants from the coastal plain region of Virginia. Virginia Agr. Exp. Sta. *Tech. Bulletin,* 123.

556. Prine, Gordon M. and G. W. Burton

    1956   The effect of nitrogen rate and clipping frequency upon the yield, protein content, and certain morphological characteristics of Coastal Bermuda grass (*Cynodon dactylon* (L.) Pers). *Agron. J.* 48(7):296-301.

557. Pritchard, G. I., W. J. Pigden and L. P. Folkins

   1964   Distribution of potassium, calcium, magnesium and so-
          dium in grasses at progressive stages of maturity. *Canad.
          J. Plant Sci.* 44:318-324.

          Nutr. Abstr., 35:1957.

          Species: Timothy and bromegrass.

558. Pyriadi, T. M., et al.

   1968   Composition and stability of pecan oils. *J. Am. Oil Chem-
          ists' Soc.* 45:437-440.

Q

559. Quiros-Perez, Felipe and C. A. Elvehjem

   1957   Nutritive value of Quinoa proteins. *J. of Agr. and Food
          Chem.* 5(7):538-541.

R

560. Rabideau, G. S. and M. B. Edwards

   1951   Nitrogen and amino-acid content of the various parts of
          Andropogon ischaemum L. *Plant. Physiol.* 26:798-806.

141

561. Radwan, M. A.

1969 Chemical composition of the sapwood of four tree species in relation to feeding by the black bear. *For. Sci.* 15(1): 11-16.

Analysis of the contents of sugars, nitrogen and mineral elements, and the kinds of sugars and soluble nitrogenous compounds in sapwood of 20-30 yr. old trees of *Pseudotsuga menziesii* (Mirb) Franco, *Tsuga heterophylla* (Raf.) Sarg., *Thuja plicata* Donn, and *Alnus rubra* Bong. Minerals: P, Ca, Mg, Fe and Mn.

562. Rashidov, T. R. and N. Akundzhanov

1971 Poluchenie vysobobelkovykk form kukuruzy pri gibridizatsii ee s teosinte. [Acquiring a high albumin form of corn by hybridizing it with teosinte]. *S-KH Biol.* 6(2): 305-308.

The content of raw protein in the endosperm of teosinte was 19.6-27.9 percent.

Species: *Zea mexicana.*

563. Rauzi, Frank, L. I. Painter and L. Landers

1965 Blue grama holds nutrients. *The Wyoming Stockman Farmer* 71(8):62.

564. Rauzi, Frank, L. I. Painter and A. K. Dobrenz

1969 Mineral and protein contents of blue grama and western wheatgrass. *J. Range Mgmt.* 22(1):47-49.

Crude protein, K, P, Mn, Mg, Fe, Cu, Zn and Ca at various times during the growing season.

Species: *Bouteloua gracilis; Agropyron smithii.*

565. Reifsnyder, William E.

1961   Seasonal variation in the moisture content of the green leaves of mountain laurel. *For. Sci.* 7(1):16-23.

Analysis done on old-growth and new-growth. 1. Leaves of plants on rocky shallow soil are drier than those of plants on deeper soils. 2. Old-growth displays cyclical variation of H_2O content: min: May, Max: late summer. 3. No relationship between moisture content and dryness of month; and 4. New leaves (300%) decrease steadily approaching previous year's leaves asymptotically (in 2 months time).

Species: *Kalmia latifolia* L.

566. Reuther, W., T. W. Embleton and W. W. Jones

1958   Mineral nutrition of tree crops. *Annual Rev. Plant Phys.* 9:175-206.

Comprehensive survey of lit. up to 1957 for work done on the nutritional mineral requirements of fruit trees.

567. Reveron, R., A. J. de J. Montilla and A. Funes

1967   Preliminary investigations of the forage characteristics of *Gliricidia sepium. Zootec. Vet.* 22:36-44. Spanish.

Nutr. Abstr., 37:6085.

Proximate analysis reported.

568. Reynolds, H. G.

1967   Chemical constituents and deer use of some crown sprouts in Arizona chaparral. *J. Forestry* 65(12):905-908.

Monthly precipitation and temperature, and monthly

Reynolds, H. G. (cont.)

crude pretein, crude fiber, moisture, Ca and P content of crown sprouts of 3 species reported along with a comparison of crude protein to moisture content, and analysis of monthly utilization as browse.

Species: *Cercocarpus betuloides* Nutt., *Quercus turbinella* Greene, *Garrya wrightii* Torr.

569. Reynolds, H. G. and A. W. Sampson

1943 Chaparral crown sprouts as browse for deer. *J. Wildl. Mgmt.* 7:119-123.

Analyzed for silica-free ash, Ca, P, Ca: P ratio, crude protein, crude fiber, moisture: analysis divided into young crown sprouts; leafy stems, full bloom; leafy stems, seeds forming; leafy stems, seeds formed. Young crown sprouts have more of everything except fiber.

Species: *Adenostoma fasciculatum.*

570. Richards, M. D. S., H. M. Sell and J. W. Thomas

1967 A study of the lipid constituents of bird's foot trefoil (*Lotus corniculatus*). *Phytochemistry* 6:303-308.

Nutr. Abstr., 38:295.

Species: *Lotus corniculatus.*

571. Richardson, C.

1889 The agricultural grasses and forage plants of the U.S.A.— The chemical composition of grasses. U.S.D.A. *Spec. Bulletin,* 133-137.

572. Riou, P., G. Delorme and F. Sylvestre

1941   De la repartition du cuivre dans les arbres a feuilles cadu-
ques du Quebec. *Ann Assn. Can. Fran. Avanc. Sci.* 7:73.

573. —.

1942   Variations de la teneur en cendres et en cuivre des organes
decidus de quelques arbes, au cours d'une annee. *Ann
Assn. Can. Fran. Avanc. Sci.* 8:77.

574. Roberts, E. N.

1926   Wyoming forage plants and their chemical composition.
Studies No. 7. Wyoming Agr. Exp. Sta. *Bulletin*, 146:35-
39.

575. Robertson, J. H. and C. Torrel

1958   Phenology as related to chemical composition of plants
and to cattle gains on summer ranges in Nevada. Neveda
Agr. Exp. Sta. *Tech. Bulletin*, 197, 38 pp.

576. Robinson, W. O. and G. Edgington

1942   Boron content of hickory and some other trees. *Soil Sci.*
53:309-312.

577. —.

1945   Minor elements in plants and some accumulator plants.
Soil Sci. 60:15-28.

A review of the literature (40 refs.) as well as a report on
some new data. Al_2O_3, SiO_2, Fe_2O_3, Mn O, Ca O, Mg O,
K_2O, Na_2O, P_2O_5, rate earth elements, As, Zn, Ba, B,
Co, Cu, F, I, Mo, Se and V_2O_5.

145

578. —.

    1948   Toxic aspect of molybdenum in vegetation. *Soil Sci.* 66: 197-198.

    Mo O_3 contents (ppm) of 50 samples of various species.

579. Rogers, David J.

    1959   Cassava leaf protein. *Econ. Bot.* 13:261-263.

    Amino acid analyses.

    Species: *Manihot esculentus.*

580. Rogers, L. H., D. E. Gall and R. M. Barnette

    1939   The zinc content of weeds and volunteer grasses and planted land covers. *Soil Sci.* 47:237-244.

581. Rotar, P. P.

    1965   Tannins and crude proteins of tick clovers (*Desmodium* spp.). *Trop. Agric.,* Trinidad 42:333-337.

    Nutr. Abstr., 36:2260.

    Twenty-three species of *Desmodium* analyzed for tannin and crude protein content.

582. Roth, Elmer P. and O. L. Copeland

    1957   Uptake of nitrogen and calcium by fertilized shortleaf pine. *J. For.* 55:281-284.

    Increased nitrogen content in needles with increased quantity of fertilizer.

583. Routley, D. G. and J. T. Sullivan

  1958 The isolation and analysis of hemicelluloses of brome
        grass. *Agr. and Food Chem.* 6:687.

584. Rovira, A. D. and J. R. Harris

  1961 Plant root excretions in relation to the rhizosphere effect.
        V. The exudation of B-group vitamins. *Plant and Soil* 14:
        119-214.

585. Ruš, V. A. and V. V. Lizunova

  1967 [Chemical composition of pine nut kernels]. *Vop. Pitan.*
        26(3):93. Russian.

        Nutr. Abstr., 38:301. (See for data).

        Proximate analysis plus fructose, sucrose, glucose, dextrin,
        starch cellulose, pentosan, lecithin, mg/100g Ca, P, Fe,
        Mg, K, Al, Si, Mn, Cu, Mo, Ni, Pb, Ag, Sr, Zn, ascorbic
        acid and carotene.

586. —.

  1969 [Major and trace elements in pine nuts]. *Vop. Pitan.*
        28(2):52-55. Russian.

        Nutr. Abstr., 39:6697.

        Pine nut samples from 1966 harvest in Siberia. Na, K, P,
        Mg, Ca, Fe, Mn, Cu, Zn, Mo, Si, Al, I, B, Ni, Co, Pb, Sr
        and Ag (mg% dry kernel).

S

587. Sakai, T., H. Maarse, R. E. Kepner, W. G. Jennings and W. M. Longhurst

1967 Volatile components of Douglas-fir needles. *J. Agric. Food. Chem.* 15(6):1070.

Species: *Pseudotsuga menziesii* (Mirb.) Franco.

588. Salgues, R.

1962 [Botanical, chemical and toxicological study of different species of *Atriplex* L. (tourn.) (Chenopodiaceae)]. *Qual. Plant. et Materiae vegetabiles* 9:71-102. French: German Summary.

Nutr. Abstr., 33:243.

Proximate analyses of various genera and species of Chenopodiaceae reported on. (5 species dealt with).

589. Sallans, H. R.

1964 Factors affecting the composition of Canadian oil-seeds. *J. Amer. Oil Chem. Soc.* 41:215-218.

Nutr. Abstr., 34:5566.

A review of the influence of various factors including climate, breeding and economics on the oil and fatty acid composition of rapeseed and linseed.

590. Salo, M. L. with T. Makinen

1965 On the content of cell-wall constituents in various plant materials. *Maataloust. Aikakousk.* 37:127-134.

Salo, M. L. with T. Makinen (cont.)

Nutr. Abstr., 36:311.

Forty-three plant materials including *Equisetum,* ferns, mosses and *Stellaria media* analyzed for hemicellulose, cellulose, mannose, pentose anhydrides, uronic anhydrides and neutral sugar anhydrides in hemicellulose.

591. Sampson, A. W. and R. Samisch

1935 Growth and seasonal changes in composition of oak leaves. *Plant Physiol.* 10:739-751.

Proximate contents of oak leaves + SiO_2, CaO, P_2O_5, K_2O, Na_2O, and Cl. Data reported in both g/1000 leaves and g/1000 in.[z]

592. Sanchez-Marroquin, A. and M. del C. Rocha

1967 [Chemical characterization of silages of maguey (*Agave atrovirens* Karw.)] . *Ciencia,* Mexico 25:169-172. Spanish: English Summary.

Nutr. Abstr., 39:351.

593. Santini, R., Jr., F. M. Berger, G. Berdasco, T. W. Sheehy, J. Aviles and I. Davila

1962 Folic acid activity in Puerto Rican foods. *J. Amer. Diet. Assn.* 41:562-567.

Nutr. Abstr., 33:4307.

Values tabulated for about 80 types of food.

594. Sauer, Jonathan D.

> 1950 The grain amaranths: A survey of their history and classi-
> fication. *Annals of the Missouri Bot. Gard.* Vol. 37, pp.
> 561-632.

595. —.

> 1957 Recent migration and evolution of the dioecious amaran-
> thus. *Evolution* Vol. 11, No. 1, pp. 11-31.

596. —.

> 1967 The grain amaranths and their relatives: A revised taxono-
> mic and geographic survey. *Annals of the Missouri Bot.*
> *Gard.* Vol. 54, No. 1, pp. 103-137.

597. Savage, D. A. and V. G. Heller

> 1947 Nutritional qualities of range forage plants in relation to
> grazing with beef cattle on the Southern Plains Experi-
> mental Range. U.S.D.A. *Tech. Bulletin,* 943, 61 pp.
>
> Species: perennial grasses (14 spp.), annual grass (1 sp.),
> palatable forbs (3 spp.), shrubs (2) analyzed on a monthly
> basis for 1 year. Proximate contents reported for Turke-
> stan bluestem, Caucasian bluestem and weeping lovegrass.
> Carotene content reported for bluegrama, buffalo grass,
> sand lovegrass, sand paspalum, sand bluestem, sand drop-
> seed and Texas bluegrass.

598. Schentzel, Dennis L.

> 1964 The carbohydrate composition and *in vitro* digestibility
> of western wheatgrass at various growing stages as de-
> termined by leaf number and cutting date. M.S. Thesis,
> South Dakota State University.

599. Schmidt, W. H. and W. L. Colville

1963   Forage yield and composition of teosinte, corn and forage sorghum grown under irrigation. *Agron. J.* 55:327-328.

Nutr. Abstr., 34:2126.

Proximate contents, carotene content, pH of silage, stem leaf ratio, dry weight of leaf and stem tissues.

600. Schneider, Burch H.

1947   Feeds of the world, their digestibility and composition. West Virginia Agr. Exp. Sta. *Bulletin,* Morgantown, 299 pp.

601. Schneiter, A. A., W. C. Whitman and K. L. Larson

1969   Sainfoin—a new legume for North Dakota? *N. Dakota Farm Res.* 27:11-13.

Nutr. Abstr., 40:4775.

Onobrychis viciaefolia-crude protein in tops from May-August declined from 34 to 9 percent.

602. Scholl, J. M.

1955   The chemical composition of yellow rocket (*Barbarea vulgaris*). *Agron. J.* 47:104-105.

Weekly samples (May-June, 1954) representing early bud stage through green seed pod stage analyzed for proximate contents, P, Ca and K.

603. Scofield, Carl S.

1940   Boron absorption by sunflower seedlings. *J. Agr. Res.*

Scofield, Carl S. (cont.)

61(1):41-56.

Boron content of leaves and stems of plants grown in solutions of known concentrations.

604. Seay, W. A. and L. E. DeMumbrum

1958 Minor element content of eight Kentucky soils and *Lespedeza. Agron. J.* 50:237-240.

Plot of the relationship of availability in soil (ppm) against content in *Lespedeza* (ppm) for Ni and Mn; 2) Mn and Ni (ppm) plotted against soil pH; 3) range of available minor elements in soils and plants for Co, Cu, Zn, Mn and Ni reported.

605. Segelquist, C. A., H. L. Short, F. D. Ward and R. G. Leonard

1972 Quality of some winter deer forages in the Arkansas Ozarks. *J. Wildl. Mgmt.* 36(1):174-177.

Percentage crude protein, cell contents, hemicellulose, lignocellulose, and the ratio of lignocellulose to lignocellulose plus hemicellulose reported.

Species: *Junipers virginiana, Acer rubrum, Cornus florida, Vaccinium vacillans, V. stamineum, Fraxinus* spp., *Prunus* spp., *Amelanchier canadensis*, dead oak leaves, sedges and grasses.

606. Seigler, D. S., K. L. Mikolajczak, C. R. Smith, Jr. and I. A. Wolff

1970 Structure and reactions of a cyanogenetic lipid from *Cordia verbenacea* DC. seed oil. *Chem. Phys. Lipids* 4(2):147-161.

152

Seigler, D. S., K. L. Mikolajczak, C. R. Smith, Jr. and I. A. Wolff (cont.)

Boraginaceae.

607. Selik, M. and H. Zeigler

1969   Der Zucket-, Eiweiss-und Vitamingehalt des Beerenzapfensaftes von *Juniperus drupacea* Labill ("Andiz pekmezi"). [The sugar, protein and vitamin content of the "berries" of *Juniperus drupacea* Labill. ("Andiz pekmezi")]. *Qual. Plant. Materiae Vegetabiles* 17:265-272. German: English Summary.

Nutr. Abstr., 40:4792.

Mash from the strobile used in Turkey, Syria and Macedonia called Andiz pekmezi is analyzed.

608. Sheldon, R. M., R. C. Lindsay and L. M. Libbey

1972   Identification of volatile flavor compounds from roasted filberts. *J. Food Sci.* 37(2):313-316.

Nutr. Abstr., 42:8018.

609. Sherrod, L. B.

1971   Nutritive value of *Kochia scoparia*. I. Yield and chemical composition of three stages of maturity. *Agron. J.* 63(2): 343-344.

Nutr. Abstr., 42:374.

Proximate analysis.

Species: *Kochia scoparia* (L.) Schrod.

610. Shipley, M. A. and F. B. Headley

> 1948   Nutritive value of wild meadow hay as affected by time of cutting. Nev. Agr. Exp. Sta. *Bulletin,* 181, 23 pp.
>
> Four year study of wire grass and sedge meadow hay clipped at 2-week intervals. Early-cut hay nutritionally superior to late-cut hay.

611. Short, Henry L. and A. Harrell

> 1969   Nutrient analysis of two browse species. *J. Range Mgmt.* 22(1):40-43.
>
> Proximate contents of current and old twigs, leaves and fruit (*Callicarpa* only), plus cell wall content, cell content, acid detergent fiber, acid detergent lignin and cellulose.
>
> Species: *Callicarpa americana, Viburnum rufidulum.*

612. Sidhu, K. S. and W. H. Pfander

> 1968   Metabolic inhibitor(s) in orchardgrass (*Dactylis glomerata* L.). *J. Dairy Sci.* 51:1042-1045.
>
> Nutr. Abstr., 39:346.

613. Siminovitch, D., C. M. Wilson and D. R. Briggs

> 1953   Studies on the chemistry of the living bark of black locust in relation to frost hardiness. V. Seasonal transformations and variations in the carbohydrates: starch-sucrose inter-conversions. *Plant Physiol.* 28:383-400.

614. Sims, Phillip L., G. R. Lovell and D. Hervey

> 1971   Seasonal trends in herbage and nutrient production of important sandhill grasses. *J. Range Mgmt.* 24:55-59.

154

615. Sims, R. P. A.

1971   Edible protein products from cruciferae seed meals. *J. Amer. Oil Chem. Soc.* 48(11):733-736.

Nutr. Abstr., 42:8015.

616. Singh, C. P. and S. K. Talapatra

1963   Yield, chemical composition and nutritive value of the legume *Melilotus indicus* All. *Indian J. Vet. Sci.* 33:63-70.

Nutr. Abstr., 34:2140.

617. Singh, Dilbagh and E. B. Smalley

1969   Nitrogenous compounds in the xylem sap of *Ulmus americana:* Seasonal variations in relation to dutch elm disease susceptibility. *For. Sci.* 15(3):299-304.

Long column chromatograms of acidic, basic and neutral amino acids and amides as well as ammonia, gamma-amino-n-butyric acid in xylem sap of Ulmus. Also, plots of seasonal variation in proline, aline, threonine, serine and gamma-amino-n-butyric acid, ammonia and ethanolamine in xylem sap expressed as u moles/10 ml. and as percent total.

618. Sinnott, E. W.

1918   Factors determining character and distribution of food reserves in woody plants. *Bot. Gaz.* 66:162-175.

619. Slaukis, V., V. C. Runeckles and G. Krotkov

1964   Metabolites liberated by roots of white pine (*Pinus strobus* L.) seedlings. *Physiol. Plant.* 17:301-313.

Slaukis, V., V. C. Runeckles and G. Krotkov (cont.)

Occurrence of sugars, amides and organic acids in the root exudate of 9-month-old seedlings.

620. Smart, W. W. G., Jr., et al.

1960 The study of the comparative composition and digestibility of cane forage (*Arundinaria* sp.). North Carolina Agr. Exp. Sta. *Tech. Bulletin,* No. 140, 8 pp.

621. Smith, A. D.

1950 Sagebrush as a winter feed for deer. *J. Wildl. Mgmt.* 14(3):285-289.

Proximate composition and digestibility by mule deer of subsp. *typica* (big sage) reported. *Artemisia tridentata nova* (black sage) not eaten although offered to deer.

622. —.

1952 Digestibility of some native forages for mule deer. *J. Wildl. Mgmt.* 16(3):309-312.

Proximate analysis and digestibility.

Species: *Purshia tridentata* (bitter brush), *Cercocarpus ledifolius* (curl leaf mahagony), *Juniperus utahensis.*

623. —.

1957 Nutritive value of some browse plants in winter. *J. Range Mgmt.* 10(4):162-164.

Percent proximate analysis and digestibility of *Cercocarpus montanus, Cowania stansburiana, Prunus virginiana* var. *melanocarpa, Quercus gambelii, Juniperus utahensis.*

Smith, A. D. (cont.)

Table of digestible nutrients (lbs/100 lbs.) compared with nutrients in some common livestock feeds. Sagebrush, common millet hay, Timothy hay, milostores, field rea straw, sudangrass straw, bunchgrass hay, alfalfa hay, oak and corn husks.

624. Smith, C. R., Jr.

1966   Keto fatty acids from *Cuspidaria pterocarpa* seed oils. *Lipids* 1(4):268-273.

625. —.

1970   Occurrence of unusual fatty acids in plants. *Progr. Chem. Fats Other Lipids* 11(pt. 1):137-177.

626. Smith, C. R., Jr. and I. A. Wolff

1966   Glycolipids of *Briza spicata* seed. *Lipids* 1(2):123-127.

627. Smith, C. R., Jr., J. E. Hagemann and I. A. Wolff

1964   The occurrence of 6, 9, 12, 15-octadecatetraenoic acid in *Echium plantagineum* seed oil. *J. Am. Oil Chemists' Soc.* 41(4):290-291.

628. Smith, C. R., Jr., K. F. Koch and I. A. Wolff

1959   Isolation of vernolic acid from *Vernonia anthelmintica* oil. *J. Amer. Oil Chemists' Soc.* 36(5):219-220.

629. Smith, C. R., Jr., L. H. Niece, H. F. Zobel and I. A. Wolff

1964   Glycosidic constituents of *Ipomoea parasitica* seed. *Phytochemistry* 3(2):289-299.

630. Smith, C. R., Jr., M. C. Shekleton, I. A. Wolff and Q. Jones

   1959   Seed protein sources—amino acid composition and total protein content of various plant seeds. *Econ. Bot.* 13(2): 132-150.

631. Smith, C. R., Jr., M. O. Bagby, R. L. Lohmar, C. A. Glass and I. A. Wolff

   1960   The epoxy acids of *Chrysanthemum coronarium* and *Clarkia elegans* seed oils. *J. Org. Chem.* 25(2):218-222.

632. Smith, C. R., Jr., M. O. Bagby, T. K. Miwa, R. L. Lohmar and I. A. Wolff

   1960   Unique fatty acids from *Limnanthes douglasii* seed oil: The C_{20}-and C_{22}-monenes. *J. Org. Chem.* 25(10):1770-1774.

633. Smith, C. R., Jr., R. Kleiman and I. A. Wolff

   1968   *Caltha palustris* L. seed oil. A source of four fatty acids with *Cis*-5-unsaturation. *Lipids* 3(1):37-42.

634. Smith, C. R., Jr., R. M. Friedinger, J. W. Hagemann, G. F. Spencer and I. A. Wolff

   1969   *Teucrium depressum* seed oil: a new source of fatty acids with Δ^5-unsaturation. *Lipids* 4(6):462-465.

635. Smith, C. R., Jr. and R. W. Miller

   1965   A C_{26}-keto-acid from the oil of *Cuspidaria*. *Chem. Ind.* (London) 46:1910.

636. Smith, C. R., Jr., T. L. Wilson and K. L. Mikolajczak

1961 Occurrence of malvalic, sterculic and dihydrosterculic acids together in seed oils. *Chem. and Ind.* (London) 8:256-257.

637. Smith, C. R., Jr., T. L. Wilson, R. B. Bates and C. R. Scholfield

1962 Densipolic acid: a unique hydroxydienoic acid from *Lesquerella densipila* seed oil. *J. Org. Chem.* 27(9):3112-3117.

638. Smith, C. R., Jr., T. L. Wilson, T. K. Miwa, H. Zobel, R. L. Lohmar and I. A. Wolff

1961 Lesquerolic acid. A new hydroxy acid from *Lesquerella* seed oils. *J. Org. Chem.* 26(8):2903-2905.

639. Smith, E. F. and V. A. Young

1959 The effect of burning on the chemical composition of little bluestem. *J. Range Mgmt.* 12(3):139-140.

Proximate analysis of plants grown on both burned and non-burned pasture.

Species: *Andropogon scoparius.*

640. Smith, F. H., K. C. Beeson and W. E. Price

1956 Chemical composition of herbage browsed by deer in two wildlife management areas. *J. Wildl. Mgmt.* 20(4):359-367.

Comparison on a dry matter basis of proximate contents, Ca, P, Fe, Mn, Cu and Co during four seasons for various species.

159

641. Smith, Margaret Cammack and E. B. Stanley

1938 The vitamin A value of blue grama range grass at different stages of growth. *J. Agr. Res.* 56:69-71.

Method: rat growth.

Conclusion: Young grass is a potent source of vitamin A., Vitamin A value of grass decreases with age.

Species: *Bouteloua gracilis.*

642. Smith, W. H.

1965 Seasonal growth and nitrogen accumulation by loblolly pine (*Pinus taeda* L.) saplings. Ph.D. Dissertation, Miss. State Univ., Stage College. Microfilm 54-8345. University Microfilms, Inc., Ann Arbor, Michigan.

643. Smith, W. H., G. L. Switzer and L. E. Nelson

1970 Development of the shoot system of young loblolly pine: I. apical growth and nitrogen concentration. *For. Sci.* 16(4):483-490.

Monthly comparisons of foliage, bark and wood of the current flushes and of older foliage in 3 crown portions as well as similar comparisons of branch bark, branch wood and stemwood for nitrogen content (percent).

644. Smith, William H.

1969 Release of organic materials from the roots of tree seedlings. *For. Sci.* 15(2):138-143.

Micrograms released per seedling during 10-day growth period of fructose, glucose, rhamnose, sucrose, the amino acids alanine, asparagine, aspartic acid, glycine, leucine/isoleucine, methionine, phenylalanine, serine, theronine,

160

Smith, William H. (cont.)

tyrosine, and gamma-aminobutyric acid. Also, the organic acids acetic, fumaric, glycolic, malonic, oxalic and succinic acid.

645. Snyder, W. A.

1961   A chemical analysis of thirteen major deer forage plants from the Guadalupe Mountains of New Mexico and their adequacy for maintaining deer. New Mexico State University. M.S. Thesis. 58 pp.

Includes analysis of *Phoradendron juniperinum*, a mistletoe.

646. Sosulski, F. W. and J. K. Patterson

1961   Correlations between digestibility and chemical constituents of selected grass varieties. *Agron. J.* 53(3):145-149.

1)   orchard grass (6 strains), lignin-parts and total plants at 5 stages of growth.
2)   brome grass (4 strains)-lignin content of entire plant.
3)   intermediate wheatgrass (3 strains)-mean % lignin content of entire plant, leaves, stems and heads at 5 stages of growth.
4)   percentage lignin in 6 strains of crested wheatgrass (flowering stage).

647. Sotola, Jerry

1940   The chemical composition and apparent digestibility of nutrients in crested wheatgrass harvested in three stages of maturity. *J. Agr. Res.* 61(4):303-311.

Proximate contents, Ca and P reported for both fresh and water-free samples.

Species: *Agropyron cristatum* (L.) Beauv.

161

648. —.

1941   The chemical composition and apparent digestibility of nutrients in smooth brome grass harvested in three stages of maturity. *J. Agr. Res.* 63(7):427-432.

Proximate contents, Ca and P as well as digestibility reported.

Species: *Bromus inermis* Leyss.

649. Specht, A. W.

1960   Evidence for and some of the implications of a variation control mechanism in plant composition. *Soil Sci.* 89:83-91.

650. Spencer, G. F., R. Kleiman, F. R. Earle and I. A. Wolff

1969   *Cis*-5-monoenoic fatty acids of *Carlina* (Compositae) seed oils. *Lipids* 4(2):99-101.

651. —.

1970   Unusual olefinic fatty acids in seed oils from two genera in the Ranunculaceae. *Lipids* 5(2):277-278.

Four out of five species of *Ranunculus* had oil with 2 to 4% *Cis*-7-, *Cis*-10-hexadecadienoic acid. *Anemone* spp: 0 to 20% gamma-linolenic acid depending upon species.

In both genera, linoleic and linolenic acids were major components.

652. —.

1970   The *Trans*-6 fatty acids of *Picramnia sellowii* seed oil. *Lipids* 5(3):285-287.

653. Spencer, G. F., R. Kleiman, R. W. Miller and F. R. Earle

    1971   Occurrence of *Cis*-6-hexadecenoic acid as the major component of *Thunbergia alata* seed oil. *Lipids* 6(10):712-714.

654. Spinner, George P. and J. S. Bishop

    1950   Chemical analysis of some wildlife foods in Connecticut. *J. Wildl. Mgmt.* 14(2):175-180.

           Proximate analyses of seeds, fruits, pods, berries and capsules of approximately 140 genera and species tabulated. Comparison of Fall and Winter seeds and fruits indicated differences resulting from seasonality not significant.

655. Sprague, V. G. and J. T. Sullivan

    1950   Reserve carbohydrates in orchard grass clipped periodically. *Plant Physiol.* 25:92-102.

656. Squibb, Robert L., E. J. Braham and N. S. Scrimshaw

    1957   Utilization of the carotenoids of bamboo leaves, teosinte and ixbut by New Hampshire chicks. *Poultry Sci.* 6: 1241-1244.

           Analysis of dehydrated forage: ash, Ca, Fe, P, moisture, ether extract, crude fiber, N, carotene, Vitamins B_2, B_3, C and Niacin.

           Species: Ixbut = *Euphorbia lancifolia* (used 6-inch plant tips), teosinte = *Zea mexicana* (used whole plants 12 inches in height), yellow bamboo = *Bambusa vulgaris* (used leaves), green bamboo = *Bambusa ventricosa* (used leaves).

657. Stanley, E. B. and C. W. Hodgson

    1938   Seasonal changes in the chemical composition of some important Arizona range grasses. Arizona Agr. Exp. Sta. *Tech. Bulletin,* 73, 449-466.

658. —.

    1938   Seasonal changes in the chemical composition of some Arizona range grasses. Arizona Agr. Exp. Sta. *Tech. Bulletin,* 73, pp. 451-466.

            Proximate contents, Ca and P.

            Species: *Bouteloua gracilis, B. hirsuta, Hilaria belanger.*

659. Stanton, W. R.

    1966   The chemical composition of some tropical food plants. 6. Durian. *Trop. Sci.* 8:6-10.

            Nutr. Abstr., 37:302.

            Species: *Durio zibethinus* Murr.

660. Steinbeck, Klaus

    1965   Variations in the foliar mineral content of five widely separated seedlots of Scotch Pine. Michigan Agr. Exp. Sta. *Quarterly Bulletin,* 48, 94-100.

661. Stinson, E. E., C. J. Dooley, J. M. Purcell and J. S. Ard

    1967   Quebrachitol—a new component of maple sap and sirup. *J. Agr. Food Chem.* 15:394-397.

            Nutr. Abstr., 38:305.

662. Stoddart, L. A.

1941   Chemical composition of *Symphoricarpos rotundifolius* as influenced by soil, site, and date of collection. *J. Agr. Res.* 63(12):727-739.

Proximate contents, Ca, P and Mg.

663. Stoddart, L. A. and J. E. Greaves

1942   The composition of summer range plants in Utah. Utah Agr. Exp. Sta. *Bulletin,* 305, 22 pp.

664. Stoller, E. W. and E. J. Weber

1970   Lipid constituents of some common weed seeds. *J. Agric. Food Chem.* 18:361.

Fifteen species of *Compositae. Solanaceae, Malvaceae, Convolvulaceae, Gramineae, Amaranthaceae* and *Polygonaceae* analyzed.

665. Stone, E. L. and G. Baird

1956   Boron level and boron toxicity in red and white pine. *J. For.* 54:11-12.

666. Stone, E. L. and G. M. Will

1965   Boron deficiency in *Pinus radiata* and *P. pinaster. For. Sci.* 11(4):425-433.

ppm Boron in needles.

667. Sullivan, J. T.

1962   Evaluation of forage crops by chemical analysis. A critique. *Agron. J.* 54(6):511-515.

668. Sullivan, J. T.

1966 Studies of the hemicelluloses of forage plants. *J. Animal Sci.* 25:83-86.

Nutr. Abstr., 36:5894.

Species: hemicellulose and lignin reported (percent dry wt.) for orchard grass, brome grass, timothy, reed canary grass, Kentucky bluegrass, Kentucky 31 fescue and alfalfa.

669. Sullivan, J. T. and D. G. Routley

1955 The relationship of the protein content of forage grasses to the earliness of flowering. *Agron. J.* 47(5):206-207.

670. Sullivan, J. T. and R. J. Garber

1947 Chemical composition of pasture plants with some reference to the dietary needs of grazing animals. Pennsylvania Agr. Exp. Sta. *Bulletin,* 305, 22 pp.

671. Sullivan, J. T., T. G. Phillips and D. G. Routley

1960 Grass hemicelluloses, water-soluble hemicelluloses of grass holocellulose. *J. Agric. Food Chem.* 8(2):152.

Determinations for orchard grass, reed canary grass, tall fescue grass, timothy and Kentucky bluegrass.

672. Sullivan, J. T., T. G. Phillips, M. E. Loughlin and V. G. Sprague

1956 Chemical composition of some forage grasses. II. Successive cuttings during the growing season. *Agron. J.* 48(1): 11-14.

Species: Alta fescue, brome, Kentucky blue, orchard,

166

Sullivan, J. T., T. G. Phillips, M. E. Loughlin and V. G. Sprague (cont.)

reed canary, red top, timothy and tall oat. Protein, lignin, cellulose, crude fiber, ether extract, soluble ash and moisture content.

673. Sullivan, J. T. and V. G. Sprague

1949 The effect of temperature on the growth and composition of the stubble and roots of perennial ryegrass. *Plant Physiol.* 24(4):706-719.

Analysis of leaves, stubble and roots of plants grown in control chambers for percentage of soluble matter, reducing sugars, sucrose, fructosan, cellulose, pentosan, lignin, soluble N, insoluble N, total N, crude ash, Ca and P.

674. Swain, T. and W. E. Hillis

1959 The phenolic constituents of *Prunus domestica.* I. The quantiative analysis of phenolic constituents. *J. Sci. Food Agric.* 10:63.

675. Swank, W. G.

1956 Protein and phosphorous content of browse as an influence on southwestern deer herd levels. *Trans. 21st N.A. Wildlf. Conf.* 21:141-158.

Moisture, phosphorous and protein content of browse samples collected during April, July, January and March of 1954-1955, in various parks of the Prescott and Pinal Mt. areas of Arizona.

Species: Skunk-bush, Turbinella oak (*Q.turbinella*) Emory oak, mountain mahogany (*Cercocarpus* sp.), *Garrya wrightii,* desert ceanothus, *Arctostaphylos pungens, A.*

167

Swank, W. G. (cont.)

pringlei, Holly-leaf buckthorn, sugar sumac (*Rhus* sp.), Utah juniper and cliff-rose.

676. —.

1956 Nutrient analysis of chaparral browse species. Arizona Game and Fish Dept. Wildl. Restoration Div., Proj. W-71-R-3, WP4, J1 and 2, 15 pp (processed).

677. Swift, R. W.

1957 The nutritive evaluation of forages. Pennsylvania Agr. Exp. Sta. *Bulletin,* 615, 34 pp.

678. Swift, R. W., et al.

1952 Further determinations of the nutritive values of forages. *J. Animal Sci.* 11:389-399.

Proximate analysis of Kentucky bluegrass, Ladino clover, orchard grass (6 cutting dates), brome grass (2 cuttings), and timothy hay (3 cuttings) reported; digestibility of proximate constituents determined as well as metabolizable energy, digestible energy, digestible dry matter and total digestible nutrients. Sheep used for this determination.

679. Swift, R. W., R. L. Cowan, R. H. Ingram, K. K. Maddy, G. P. Barron, E. C. Grose and J. B. Washko

1950 The relative nutritive value of Kentucky bluegrass, timothy, brome grass, orchard grass, and alfalfa. *J. Animal Sci.* 9(3):363-372.

Proximate contents of samples collected over a period of months reported.

168

680. Switzer, G. L. and L. E. Nelson

1956 The effect of fertilization on seedling weight and utilization of N, P, and K by loblolly pine (*Pinus taeda* L.) grown in the nursery. *Proc. Amer. Soil Sci. Soc.* 20:404-408.

With no fertilizer N conc. in foliage was 1.33 percent fertilizer rate of 300 lbs/acre = 0.18 percent (added as phosphate calculated as P_2O_5).

T

681. Tahiri-Zagret, M.

1970 [Study of the amino acids of *Cyperus esculentus* for its nutritive value in weaning foods.] *Bull. Soc. Pathol. exot.* 63:279-286. French: English Summary.

Nutr. Abstr., 41:4966.

Proximate and amino acid analysis, Ca and P.

682. Taira, H.

1968 Amino acid composition of different varieties of foxtail millet (*Setaria italica*). *J. Agric. Food Chem.* 16:1025-1027.

Nutr. Abstr., 39:4581.

683. Taira, H. and H. Taira

1964 [Amino acid composition of seeds and nuts]. *J. Jap. Soc. Food Nutrition* 17:244-247. Japanese: English

169

Taira, H. and H. Taira (cont.)

Summary.

Nutr. Abstr., 35:3656.

Analysis covers many New World species.

684. Tallent, W. H.

1972 Crambe. Northern Mkt., Nutr. Res. Div., U.S. Agri. Res. Serv., CA-71-36, 4 pp.

685. Tallent, W. H., J. Harris, I. A. Wolff and R. E. Lundin

1966 (R)-13-hydroxy-Cis-9-Trans-11-octadecadienoic acid, the principal fatty acid from *Coriaria nepalensis* Wall. seed oil. *Tetrahedron Letters* (36):4329-4334.

686. Tamm, C. O.

1955 Studies on forest nutrition I. Seasonal variation in the nutrient content of conifer needles. *Medd. Fran Statens Skogsforskninst.* 45, Nr. 5, 34 pp.

687. Tamm, Carl Olof

1956 Studies on forest nutrition III. The effect of supply of plant nutrients to a forest stand on a poor site. *Meddelanden Fran Statens Skogsforsknings Institut.* 46:1-84. English Summary.

Pinus sylvestris L. Fertilized with nitrogen at varying rates of 0-200 kg/ha. best diameter growth was related to a foliage concentration of 2.0-2.5% N.

688. Tannous, R. I. and M. Ullah

> 1969 Effects of autoclaving on nutritional factors in legume seeds. *Trop. Agric.,* Trinidad 46:123-129.
>
> Nutr. Abstr., 39:6678.
>
> Species: *Cicer arietinum* chick peas; *Lupinus terminus* lupins.

689. Taylor, F. H.

> 1956 Variation in sugar content of maple sap. Vermont Agric. Exp. Sta. *Bulletin,* 587. Burlington, Vermont.

690. Taylor, J. R. and E. Fernandez-Flores

> 1969 Chemical composition of fresh elderberries. *J. Assn. Off. Anal. Chem.* 52:643-646.
>
> Nutr. Abstr., 40:285.
>
> Proximate analysis; other analyses.
>
> Species: *Sambucus nigra.*

691. Tew, Ronald K.

> 1970 Seasonal variation in the nutrient content of Aspen foliage. *J. Wildl. Mgmt.* 34(2):475-478.
>
> Nutr. Abstr., 41:2458.
>
> Protein, ash, fat, H_2O, Ca, P, Ca/P, K, Mg and Na.
>
> Species: *Populus tremuloides.*

692. Thomas, W.

 1945   Present status of diagnosis of mineral requirements of plants by means of leaf analysis. *Soil Sci.* 59:353.

693. Thorsland, O. A.

 1967   Nutritional analyses of selected deer foods in South Carolina. *Proc. S.C. Assn. Game and Fish Comm. Conf.* 20: 84-104.

694. Tolbert, N. E. and H. Wiebe

 1955   Phosphorous and sulphur compounds in plant xylem sap. *Plant Physiol.* 30:499-504.

695. Tomlin, D. G., R. R. Johnson and B. A. Dehority

 1965   Relationship of lignification to *in vitro* cellulose digestibility of grasses and legumes. *J. Anim. Sci.* 24:161.

696. Tookey, H. L. and H. S. Gentry

 1969   Proteinase of *Jarilla chocola,* a relative of papaya. *Phytochemistry* 8(6):989-991.

697. Tookey, H. L. and Q. Jones

 1965   New sources of water-soluble seed gums. *Econ. Bot.* 19(2):165-174.

         Seeds from 300 species of 139 genera in 31 plant families surveyed for water-soluble gum (Mucilage). Four families Leguminosae, Plantaginaceae, Cruciferae and Convolvulaceae have species whose seeds contain more than 18% gum.

Tookey, H. L. and Q. Jones (cont.)

Tables list gum, % of air dried seed (N-free and crude), nature of gum, weight of seed/1000 and growth habit of plant for all plants surveyed.

698. Tookey, H. L., R. L. Lohmar, I. A. Wolff and Q. Jones

1962 New sources of seed mucilages. *J. Agric. Food Chem.* 10(2):131-133.

Twenty legumes reported: seed mucilage content (%) and mucilage purification, composition (%) and optical rotation of galactomannans for these. Table of seed mucilage distribution by family (175 species in 26 families surveyed).

699. Tookey, H. L. and S. G. Yates

1972 The alkaloids of tall fescue: Loline (Festucine) and Perloline. *An. Quim.* 68(5-6):921-935.

Eleven alkaloids in tall fescue, *Festuca arundinacea* Schreb. similar to those in ryegrass (*Lolium perenne* L.).

700. Tookey, H. L. and T. F. Clark

1965 Evaluation of seed galactomannans from *Cassia* species as paper additives. *Tappi* 48(11):625-626.

701. Tookey, H. L., V. F. Pfeifer and C. R. Martin

1963 Gums separated from *Crotolaria intermedia* and other leguminous seeds by dry milling. *J. Agri. Food Chem.* 11(4):317-321.

702. Torgerson, Oliver and W. H. Pfander

1971 Cellulose digestibility and chemical composition of Missouri deer foods. *J. Wildl. Mgmt.* 35(2):221-231.

Cellulose content and 24 hr. *in vitro* digestibility of 35 air dried plants (Summer and Winter foods). Also, proximate chemical analysis and Ca, P and K content (air-dried basis) for 33 Summer and Winter deer food species.

703. Treichler, R., R. W. Stow and A. L. Nelson

1946 Nutrient content of some winter foods of ruffed grouse. *J. Wildl. Mgmt.* 10(1):12-17.

Gross energy (cal/gm) and proximate analyses (fresh and moisture-free).

Species: *Alnus* sp. (catkins), *Amelanchier canadensis* (buds) *Betula lutea* (buds), *Corylus rostrata* (catkins), *Epigaea repens* (leaves), *Galax aphylla* (leaves), *Gaultheria procumbens* (leaves), *Kalmia latifolia* (leaves and flower buds), *Menziesia pilosa* (buds), *Mitchella repens* (leaves), *Polystichum acrostichoides* (leaves), *Prunella vulgaris* (leaves), *Rosa humilis* (fruit), *Rumex acetosella* (leaves), and *Smilax glauca* (leaves and fruit).

704. Trelease, S. F., A. A. DiSomma and A. L. Jacobs

1960 Seleno-amino acid found in *Astragalus bisulcatus. Science* 132(3427):618.

705. Trlica, M. J., Jr. and C. W. Cook

1971 Defoliation effects on carbohydrate reserves of desert species. *J. Range Mgmt.* 24(6):418-425.

Tabulation of the following data: Average total available CHO (mg/g) reserves stored at time of fall quiescence in

Trlica, M. J., Jr. and C. W. Cook (cont.)

the roots and crowns of various species given 5 defoliation treatments (including an untreated control group) over a 3-year period.

Species: *Artemisia tridentata, A. arbuscula var. nova, Atriplex confertifolia, A. falcata, Eurotia lanata, Oryzopsis hymenoides, Stipa comata,* and *Sitanion hystrix.*

706. Trowbridge, P. F., L. D. Haigh and C. R. Moulton

1915   Studies of the timothy plant. Pt. II. The changes in the chemical composition of the timothy plant during growth and ripening, with a comparative study of the wheat plant. Missouri Agr. Exp. Sta. Res. *Bulletin, 20.*

707. Turner, B. L. and J. B. Harborne

1967   Distribution of canavanine in the plant kingdom. *Phytochemistry* (6):863-866.

Nutr. Abstr., 38:290.

Qualitative survey of legumes reported (ca. 540 species of 150 genera).

708. Tyrrell, Dorothy P., M. H. Jenkins and A. E. Weis

1951   The nutritive value of black walnuts. Missouri Agr. Exp. Sta. Res. *Bulletin,* No. 470, pp. 12.

Riboflavin, Thiamine, Niacin, Carotene, Protein and Fat analysis given.

175

709. Ullrey, D. E., et al.

    1964   Digestibility of cedar and aspen browse for the white-tailed deer. *J. Wildl. Mgmt.* 28(4):791-797.

710. —.

    1967   Digestibility of cedar and jackpine browse for the white-tailed deer. *J. Wildl. Mgmt.* 31(3):448-454.

711. —.

    1968   Digestibility of cedar and balsam fir browse for the white-tailed deer. *J. Wildl. Mgmt.* 32(1):162-171.

712. —.

    1972   Digestibility and estimated metabolizability of aspen browse for white-tailed deer. *J. Wildl. Mgmt.* 36(3):885-891.

           Proximate analysis, metabolizable energy and nitrogen balance tabulated for *Thuja* and *Populus* only.

           Species: *Thuja occidentalis* (northern white cedar), *Abies balsamea* (balsam fir), *Populus grandidentata* (large toothed aspen).

713. Underwoods, E. J.

    1965   *Trace Elements in Human and Animal Nutrition,* New York: Academic Press, Inc., 430 pp.

714. United States Department of Agriculture

Bulletins 572 and 549: Summaries on composition of U.S. Foodstuffs.

715. Urness, Philip J.

1969 Nutritional analyses and *in vitro* digestibility of mistletoes browsed by deer in Arizona. *J. Wildl. Mgmt.* 33(3): 499-505.

Crude protein, Ca, P, Ca: P ratios, dry matter, acid-detergent fiber, dry matter digestibility. Annual changes given on a month-by-month basis.

Five species of *Phoradendron*, 1 species of *Arceuthobium*.

V

716. Van Camp, John

1948 The nutrient content of the foliage of certain species of minor forest vegetation. *J. For.* 46:823-826.

N, P, K, Ca, Mg, S, Fe, Zn, B, Cu, Mn, Al, Na, S and SiO_2 content of foliage expressed as a percentage of dry weight.

Species: *Adiantum pedatum, Amphicarpa bracteata, Aralia nudicaulis, Dryopteris noveboracensis, Collinsonia canadensis, Cornus florida, Hamamelis virginiana, Juniperus virginiana* (pasture and forest), *Kalmia latifolia, Comptonia peregrina, Uvularia sessilifolia, Rubus hispidus, Viburnum acerifolium* (ridge and bottom).

717. Vandermark, Jerry L., E. M. Schmutz and P. R. Ogden

1971 Effects of soils on forage utilization in the desert grassland. *J. Range Mgmt.* 24(6):431-434.

Percent various components (N, P, K, Mg, Fe, Cu, Zn, moisture, sugar and starch) for samples of blue grama and curly-mesquite from 3 desert grassland soils.

718. Van Dyne, G. M.

1962 Micro-methods for nutritive evaluation of range forages. *J. Range Mgmt.* 15:303-314.

719. Van Dyne, G. M., G. F. Payne and O. O. Thomas

1965 Chemical composition of individual range plants from the U.S. Range Station, Miles City, Montana, from 1955-1960. U.S. Atomic Energy Commission, Oak Ridge, Tennessee.

720. Van Dyne, G. M. and H. F. Heady

1965 Dietary chemical composition of cattle and sheep grazing in common on a dry foothill annual range. *J. Range Mgmt.* 18:78-86.

Proximate contents of *Aira caryophyllea, Avena barbata, Bromus mollis, B. rigidus, Daucus pusillus, Hypochaeris glabra,* and *Navarretia* spp.

721. Van Dyne, George M.

1965 Chemical composition and digestibility of plants from annual range and from pure-stand plots. *J. Range Mgmt.* 18(6):332-337.

Proximate analyses of approximately 18 plants (mostly

Van Dyne, George M. (cont.)

grasses and legumes, but others as well; table indicates whether stems, leaves, head or entire plant was analyzed).

722. —.

1968 Prediction of non-linear programming of relative chemical composition of dietary botanical components. *J. Range Mgmt.* 21(1):37-46.

Aira caryophyllea, Avena barbata, Gastridium ventricosum, Bromus spp., *Daucus pusillus, Hypochaeris glabra, Trifolium* spp.

723. Van Etten, C. H., M. E. Daxenbichler, J. E. Peters and H. L. Tookey

1966 Variation in enzymatic degradation products from the major thioglucosides of *Crambe abyssinica* and *Brassica napus* seed meals. *J. Agr. Food Chem.* 14(4):426-430.

724. Van Etten, C. H., M. E. Daxenbichler, J. E. Peters, I. A. Wolff and A. N. Booth

1965 Seed meal from *Crambe abyssinica. J. Agr. Food Chem.* 13(1):24-27.

725. Van Etten, C. H. and R. W. Miller

1963 The neuroactive factor alpha-gamma diaminobutyric acid in angiospermous seeds. *Econ. Bot.* 17(2):107-109.

Seeds from 158 species of 39 plant families examined for alpha-gamma-diaminobutyric acid. Seeds from Cruciferae and Leguminosae more apt to contain this toxic compound.

726. Van Etten, C. H., R. W. Miller, F. R. Earle, I. A. Wolff and Q. Jones

> 1961 Hydroxyproline content of seed meals and distribution of the amino acid in kernel, seed coat, and pericarp. *Agr. and Food Chem.* 9:433-435.
>
> Analysis done on 13 genera; bibliography cites a number of related articles.

727. Van Etten, C. H., R. W. Miller, I. A. Wolff and Q. Jones

> 1961 Amino acid composition of twenty-seven selected seed meals. *Agr. and Food Chem.* 9(1):79-82.
>
> Twenty-seven genera of 13 botanical families.

728. —.

> 1963 Amino acid composition of seeds from 200 angiosperm plant species. *Agr. and Food Chem.* 11:399-410.
>
> Seed meals of 134 plant species not previously analyzed and 66 reported earlier. Percent protein, oil, N as amino acid; amino acid analyses, including teosinte, *Portulaca oleracea*, *Crotolaria* sp., *Dalea* sp., *Desmodium* sp., *Ipomoea purpurea*, *Sicyos angulatus*, etc.

729. Van Etten, C. H., W. E. Gagne, D. J. Robbins, A. N. Booth, M. E. Daxenbichler and I. A. Wolff

> 1969 Biological evaluation of Crambe seed meals and derived products by rat feeding. *Cereal Chem.* 46(2):145-155.

730. Van Etten, C. H., W. F. Kwolek, J. E. Peters and A. S. Barclay

> 1967 Plant seeds as protein sources for food or feed. Evalua-

Van Etten, C. H., W. F. Kwolek, J. E. Peters and A. S. Barclay (cont.)

> tion based on amino acid composition of 379 species. *J. Agr. Food Chem.* 15(6):1077-1089.

> One hundred sixty-five new analyses, 214 previous analysis.

731. Van Soest, P. J. and L. A. Moore

> 1966 New chemical methods for analysis of forages for the purpose of predicting nutritive value. *Proc. 9th Int. Grassland Congr.,* 1965:783-789.

732. Van Soest, P. J. and R. H. Wine

> 1967 Use of detergents in the analysis of fibrous feeds. IV. Determination of plant cell-wall constituents. *J. Assoc. Offic. Agr. Chem.* 50:50-55.

733. Varo, P. T. and D. E. Heinz

> 1970 Volatile components of cumin seed oil. *J. Agr. Food Chem.* 18:234.

734. Vaughan, J. G. and J. S. Hemingway

> 1959 The utilization of mustards. *Econ. Bot.* 13:196.

> Unpalatable and toxic substances in *Cruciferae.*

735. Vega, A. and E. A. Bell

> 1967 alpha-amino-beta-methylamino propionic acid, a new amino acid from seeds of *Cycas circinalis. Phytochemistry* 6:759-762.

Vega, A. and E. A. Bell (cont.)

Nutr. Abstr., 38:309.

Possibly neurotoxic to higher animals.

736. Vengris, Jonas, M. Drake, W. G. Colby and J. Bart

1953 Chemical composition of weeds and accompanying crop plants. *Agron. J.* 45:213-218.

Data: N, P, K, Cu, Mg composition of 17 grassland weeds (% air-dry basis) sampled in both June and September. Chemical composition (N, P, K, Ca and Mg-%air-dry basis) of weeds from onion, corn and potato fields. Comparision of relative chemical composition of weeds grown with different companion crop plants (corn, potato, onion).

737. Ventre, Emil K., S. Byall and J. L. Catlett

1948 Sucrose, dextrose and levulose content of some domestic varieties of sorgo at different stages of maturity. *J. Agr. Res.* 76:145-151.

Data: Analysis of sorgo juices at the milk stage of maturity (dissolved solids, sucrose, purity, invert sugar, dextrose and levulose), also at the "dough-to-ripe" stage and at the "dead ripe" stage.

Species: *Sorghum vulgare* Pers.

738. Verme, L. J.

1953 Production and utilization of acorns in Clinton County, Michigan. Unpublished M.S. Thesis. Michigan State University, 77 pp.

182

739. Vidal, C. and C. Varela

1969   "Sobre el aminograma del higo chumbo y de la bellota y possibilidades de mejora de la calidad nutritiva de sus proteinas, [Aminograms of prickly pear and acorn and possibilities of improving the nutritive value of their proteins] ." *Rev. Nutricion animal,* Madrid 7:53-66. In Spanish with English Summary.

Nutr. Abstr., 40:292.

Species: *Opuntia ficus indica, Quercus ilex.*

740. Vil'jams, V. V. and N. K. Semenova

1967   [Distribution of vitamin E in plants). *Izv. Timirjazev. Sel'skohoz. Akad.* 6:36-47. Russian: English Summary.

Nutr. Abstr., 38:4598.

Values tabulated for Vit. E content on both a fresh and dry matter basis in leaves of 151 species at the time of flowering; also analyzed are 16 species, flowers and the leaves of 21 vegetables. In leaves range of tocopherols was 3.3-375.0 mg/100g dry matter.

741. Villegas, M. E., R. O. Cravioto, H. G. Massieu, G. J. Guzman and M. L. Suarez Soto

1956   Contribucion al conocimiento de los effectos de la coccion en el contenido de tiamina, riboflavina y niacina en algunos alimentos mexicanos. *Ciencia* 16:65-76. Inst. Nac. Nutriol, Mexico, D.F.

Foods were vegetables bought in the markets of Mexico City.

183

742. Vinal, H. N. and R. McKee

1916 Moisture content and shrinkage of forage and the relation of these factors to the accuracy of experimental data. U.S.D.A. *Bulletin,* 353, 21 pp.

743. Voris, LeRoy, M. F. Lawson, E. J. Thacker and W. W. Wainio

1940 Digestible nutrients of feeding stuffs for the domestic rabbit. *J. Agr. Res.* 61(9):673-683.

Proximate analyses.

Species: *Lespedeza sericea,* common Lespedeza, Kudzu hay, blue grass, Sudan grass, *Barbarea vulgaris,* orchard grass, *Geum rivale,* green sweet lupine, Darnel grass, etc.

W

744. Wainio, Walter W. and E. B. Forbes

1941 The chemical composition of forest fruits and nuts from Pennsylvania. *J. Agr. Res.* 62(10):627-635.

Proximate analysis, tannin, cellulose, lignin, Ca, Mg and P.

Species: 35 mast products from Central Pennsylvania. Species of: *Malus, Solanum, Rubus, Viburnum, Vaccinium, Prunus, Aronia, Magnolia, Aecinium, Cornus, Sambucus, Vitis, Celtis, Crataegus, Amelanchier, Sorbus, Nemopanthus, Benzoin, Rhus, Ilex, Aesculus, Castanea, Corylus, Hicoria (Carya), Quercus* (5 kinds) and *Juglans.*

Genus, species, common name, location, portion analyzed are included in the data.

745. Waite, B.

  1958   The water-soluble carbohydrates of grasses. IV. The effect of different levels of fertilizer treatments. *J. Sci. Food and Agr.* 9:39-43.

746. Walker, H. G., Jr., B. Lai, W. C. Rockwell and G. O. Kohler

  1970   Preparation and evaluation of popped grains for feed use. *Cereal Chem.* 47:513-521.

         Nutr. Abstr., 41:2404.

         Popping reduces amount of extractable protein.

747. Walker, T. W., A. F. R. Adams and H. D. Orchiston

  1955   The effects of interactions of molybdenum, lime and phosphate treatments on the yield and composition of white clover, grown on acid molybdenum-responsive soils. *Plant and Soil* 6:201-220.

748. Wasser, C. H.

  1945   High protein content makes winterfat value forage for Colorado ranges. *Colo. Farm Bulletin* 7:6, 7, 13.

         Species: *Eurotia lanata* (Chenopodiaceae).

749. Waters, N. J.

  1915   Studies of the timothy plant. Pt. I. Influence of maturity upon yield, composition, digestibility, palatability, and feeding value of timothy hay. Missouri Agr. Exp. Sta. *Res. Bulletin, 79.*

750. Watkins, James M.

1940 The growth habits and chemical composition of brome-grass, *Bromus inermis* Leyss, as affected by different environmental conditions. *Amer. Soc. Agr. J.* 32:527-538.

751. Watkins, W. E.

1939 Monthly variation in carotene content of two important range grasses. *Sporobolus flexuosus* and *Bouteloua erio-pada. J. Agr. Res.* 58:695-699.

752. —.

1943 Composition of range grasses and browse at varying stages of maturity. New Mexico Agr. Exp. Sta. *Tech. Bulletin,* 311.

753. Watkins, W. E. and J. H. Knox

1950 The relation of the carotene content of range forage to the vitamin A requirement of breeding cows. *J. Animal Sci.* 9:23-29.

(Mg/1000 gms) carotene content given for vegetative por-tion of three-awn grass (*Aristida* sp.), black grama grass (*Bouteloua eriopoda*), and for *Yucca elata* blooms.

754. Watt, B. K. and A. L. Merrill

1950 Composition of Foods—Raw, Processed, Prepared. U.S.-D.A. Handbook No. 8.

755. Watterston, K. G. and A. L. Leaf

1963 Effect of N, P, and K fertilization on yield and sugar con-

186

Watterston, K. G. and A. L. Leaf (cont.)

>tent of sap of sugar maple trees. *Soil Sci. Amer. Proc.* 27:236-238.

756. Webster, J. E., G. Shrycock and P. Cox

>1963   The carbohydrate composition of two species of grama grasses. Okla. Agr. Exp. Sta. *Tech. Bulletin* T-104, 16 pp.

757. Weems, J. B. and A. W. Hess

>1903   The chemical composition of nuts used as food. *Proc.* Iowa Academy of Sciences 10:108-111.

>Proximate analysis of almonds, brazils, filberts, hickory, pecans, walnuts, chestnuts and peanuts.

758. Weihe, H. D. and M. Phillips

>1940   Hemicelluloses of wheat straw. *J. Agr. Res.* 60:781-786.

759. —.

>1942   Hemicelluloses of cornstalks. *J. Agr. Res.* 64(7):401-406.

760. Wein, Ross W. and N. E. West

>1971   Phenology of salt desert plants near contour furrows. *J. Range Mgmt.* 24(4):299.

>Species: *Atriplex confertifolia, A. nuttallii, A. corrugata, Hilaria jamesii.*

761. Weinmann, H.

   1952   Carbohydrate reserves in grasses. pp. 655-660 in: *Proc.*
          VIth International Grassland Congress, Penn. State Uni-
          versity.

762. Welch, Tommy G.

   1968   Carbohydrate reserves of sand reedgrass under different
          grazing intensities. *J. Range Mgmt.* 21(4):216-220.

          Species: *Calamovilfa longifolia.*

763. Wells, C. G. and L. J. Metz

   1963   Variation in nutrient content of loblolly pine needles with
          season, age, soil and position on the crown. *Proc. Soil*
          Sci. Soc. Am. 27(1):90-93.

764. White, E. M.

   1972   Ponderosa pine seedling greenhouse-growth on Black Hills
          prairie and forest soils. *Soil Sci.* 114(5):406-407.

          Comparison of needle composition: Ca, K, P and N.

765. White, G. A. and F. R. Earle

   1971   *Vernonia anthelmintica:* A potential seed oil source of
          epoxy acid. IV. Effects of lime, harvest date, and seed
          storage on quantity and quality of oil. *Agron. J.* 63:441-
          443.

766. White, George A. and I. A. Wolff

   1968   From wild plants to new crops in U.S.A. *World Crops*
          20(3):70-76.

767. Whitman, W. C.

>   1941   Seasonal changes in bound water content of some prairie
>   grasses. *Bot. Gaz.* 103:38-63.
>
>   Species: Uplands: *Agropyron* sp., *Bouteloua* sp., *Stipa
>   comata.*
>   Sagebrush: *Agropyron* sp.
>   Sandgrass: *Calamovilfa* sp., *Koeleria* sp.
>   Big bluestem: *Andropogon* sp., *Stipa spartea.*

768. Whitman, W. C., D. W. Bolin, E. W. Klosterman, H. J. Klosterman, K. D. Ford, L. Moomaw, D. G. Hoag and M. L. Buchanan

>   1951   Carotene, protein, and phosphorous in range and tame
>   grasses of Western North Dakota.   North Dakota Agr.
>   Exp. Sta. *Bulletin,* 370, 55 pp.

769. Wierzchowski, Z., A. Leonowicz, K. Sapiecha and A. Sykut

>   1962   Tree leaves as a source of carotenes with provitamin activ-
>   ity. *Rocz. Nauk rol.* [B] , 81:87-102. Polish: Russian
>   and English Summary.
>
>   Nutr. Abstr., 33:5946.
>
>   Carotenes in leaves or needles were estimated throughout
>   the season in 25 species and once in August or September
>   in 74 species of exotic and native trees and in 11 herbace-
>   ous species.

770. Williams, John S.

>   1953   Seasonal trends of minerals and proteins in prairie grasses.
>   *J. Range Mgmt.* 6(2):100-108.
>
>   Effects of nitrogen and phosphorous fertilization on the
>   protein and phosphorous content of native grasses at
>   varying growth stages tabulated.

189

771. Williams, John Simeon

1949   The phosphorous, calcium and protein content of some native prairie grasses as affected by fertilization and stage of maturity. Abstr. of Dr. Thesis. Dept. of Agronomy, Univ. of Nebraska, 11 pp.

772. Williams, M. C.

1960   Effect of sodium and potassium salts on growth and oxalate content of halogeton. *Plant Physiol.* 35(4):500-505.

773. Williams, R. D.

1957   Growth and nutrition of timothy (*Phleum pratense* L.) III. Absorption and distribution of nitrogen, phosphorous and potassium during the first year of growth. *Ann. of Appl. Biol.* 45(4):664-673.

774. Wilson, A. D.

1966   The value of *Atriplex* (saltbush) and *Kochia* (blue bush) species as food for sheep. *Australian J. Agriculture Res.* 17:147-153.

775. —.

1969   A review of browse in the nutrition of grazing animals. *J. Range Mgmt.* 22:23.

Sixty-eight references.

776. Wilson, T. L., C. R. Smith, Jr. and I. A. Wolff

1962   *Lunaria* seed oil—a rich source of C_{24} fatty acids. *J. Am. Oil Chemist's Soc.* 39(2):104-105.

777. Wilson, T. L., C. R. Smith, Jr. and K. C. Mikolajczak

   1961   Characterization of cyclopropenoid acids in selected seed
         oils. *J. Am. Oil Chemist's Soc.* 38(12):696-699.

778. Wilson, T. L., T. K. Miwa and C. R. Smith, Jr.

   1960   *Cuphea llavea* seed oil, a good source of capric acid. *J.
         Am. Oil Chemist's Soc.* 37(12):675-676.

779. Winton, A. L. and K. B. Winton

   1932   *The Structure and Composition of Foods.* New York,
         N.Y., John Wiley and Sons.

780. Wittenburg, H. and K. Nehring

   1967   Alkaloid content of different samples of *Lupinus luteus,
         Lupinus angustifolius* and *Lupinus albus. Arch. Tierer-
         nahrung* 17:227-231. German: Russian and English
         summaries.

         Nutr. Abstr., 38:296.

781. Wolf, D. D.

   1967   Characteristics of stored carbohydrates in reed canary
         grass as related to management, feed value and herbage
         yield. *Storrs Agri. Exp. Sta. Bulletin,* No. 402, pp. 34.

         Nutr. Abstr., 39:340.

         Species: *Phalaris arundinacea* L.

782. Wolff, I. A. and T. K. Miwa

   1965   Effect of unusual acids on selected seed oil analyses.

191

Wolff, I. A. and T. K. Miwa (cont.)

J. Am. Oil Chemist's Soc. 42(3):208-215.

Procedural problems discussed.

783. Wolff, Ivan A. and W. F. Kwolek

1971 Lipids of the Leguminosae. In: *Chemotaxonomy of the Leguminosae,* J. B. Harbone, D. Boutler and B. L. Turner (Eds.), Chap. 6, pp. 231-255, London.

784. Wolff, M. J., M. M. MacMasters and C. E. Rist

1950 Some characteristics of the starches of three South American seeds used for food. *Cereal Chem.* 27(3):219-222.

785. Wood, A. J., M. C. Robertson and W. D. Kitts

1958 Studies on the nutritive value of refuse screenings. I. The essential amino acid content of certain weed seeds. *Canad. J. Animal Sci.* 38:47.

Amino acid content of cruciferae seeds reported on.

Species: *Brassica juncacea, B. kaber, B. napus, B. alba, Thlaspi arvense, Sysimbrium altissimum, Camelina microcarpa.*

786. Woods, Charles D. and L. H. Merrill

1899 Nuts as food. Maine Agr. Exp. Sta., 15th Annual Report, pp. 71-92.

Proximate analysis of *Amygdalus communis* (both California and European varieties of the almond), and of *Bertholletia excelsa* (Brazil nut), also of *Corylus, Carya* (pecan and hickory), *Juglans, Quercus* and *Fagus.*

787. Woods, Frank W.

1959 Nutritional aspects of wiregrass from West Florida sandhills. *J. Range Mgmt.* 12(3):141.

Species: *Aristida stricta.* Crude protein, P, Ca, Mg, K, and Na of samples from burned and unburned areas.

788. Worley, C. L.

1937 Carbohydrate changes within the needles of *Pinus ponderosa* and *Pseudotsuga taxifolia. Plant Phsyiol.* 12:755-770.

789. Wright, Jonathan W., W. A. Lemmicu and J. N. Bright

1969 Early growth of ponderosa pine ecotypes in Michigan. *For. Sci.* 15(2):121-129.

Geographic variation in foliar mineral content of ponderosa pine: N, K, P, Ca, Mg, Mn, Fe, Cu and B.

790. Wright, Thomas, Jr.

1941 A study of the fall food supply of the ring-necked pheasant and the bob-white quail in Washington County, Rhode Island. *J. Wildl. Mgmt.* 5(3):279-296.

Proximate analysis of 25 wild plant foods (seeds and fruits).

Y

791. Yang, S. P., P. Swanson, M. Caedo and H. Fox

1955 Nutritive value of proteins in teosinte grain. Amer. Inst. of Nutr., *Federation Proc.* 14:455.

792. Yermanos, D. M.

1966 Variability in seed oil composition of 43 *Linum* species. *J. Amer. Oil Chemist's Soc.* 43:546-549.

Nutr. Abstr., 37:2300.

793. Yermanos, D. M., B. H. Beard, K. S. Gill and M. P. Anderson

1966 Fatty acid composition of seed oil of wild species of *Linum. Agron. J.* 58:30-32.

794. Young, O. R. and K. K. Otagaki

1958 The variation in protein and mineral composition of Hawaii range grass and its potential effect on cattle nutrition. Hawaii Agr. Exp. Sta. *Bulletin,* 119, 27 p.

Z

795. Zimmermann, M. H.

1957a Translocation of organic substances in the phloem of trees. I. The nature of sugars in sieve tube exudate of trees. *Plant Physiol.* 32:288-291.

796. —.

    1957b Translocation, etc., II. On the translocation mechanism in the phloem of white ash (*Fraxinus americana* L.). *Plant Physiol.* 32:399-404.

Index of Scientific Plant Names
by number of entry

Index

Index

Index

200

Index

Vernonia anthelmintica 373, 628, 765

Xanthium orientale 182

Xeranthemum annuum 553

Zinnia pumila 112

Convolvulaceae 664
Ipomoea parasitica 629
I. purpurea 728

Coriariaceae
Coriaria nepalensis 685

Cornaceae
Cornus florida 57, 152, 169, 276, 312, 605, 716
C. paniculata 292
C. racemosa 14
C. stolonifera 4, 14, 216
Cornus sp. 414, 744

Corylaceae
Corylus americana 14, 152, 292
C. avellana 329
C. rostrata 237, 703
Corylus sp. 347, 608, 744, 786,

Cruciferae 9, 248, 403, 460, 467, 469, 615, 725, 734
Alyssum maritimum 448

Barbarea vulgaris 602, 743

Berteroa incana 247

Brassica alba 785
B. campestris 10, 161

B. carinata 10
B. juncacea 10, 785
B. kaber 785
B. napus 9, 10, 92, 723, 785
B. nigra 10
B. oleracea 10
Brassica sp. 501

Camelina microcarpa 785

Cardamine impatiens 449, 450

Cardaria draba var. repens 38

Crambe abyssinica 15, 159, 723, 724
Crambe sp. 160, 390, 684, 729

Lesquerella auriculata 357
L. densipila 637
L. lasiocarpa 163
Lesquerella sp. 158, 171, 366, 456, 464, 638

Lunaria sp. 776

Nasturtium sp. 241

Pastinaca sativa 404

Selenia grandis 448

Sinapis alba 10
Sinapis sp. 501

Sophia pinnata 258

Sysimbrium altissimum 785
S. pinnatum 258

Index

Index

Index

Index

Index

Hedysarum sulphurescens 335

Lespedeza bicolor 110
L. cuneata 493
L. japonica 110
L. sericea 288, 743
L. stipulacea 493
L. virginica 152
Lespedeza sp. 492, 604, 743

Lotus corniculatus 39, 43, 48,
    188, 397, 570

Lupinus albus 780
L. angustifolius 780
L. luteus 780
L. mutabilis 121
L. sericens 221
L. terminus 688
L. tricolor 121
Lupinus sp. 109, 203, 245, 380,
    743

Medicago sativa 30, 43, 48, 49,
    100, 102, 143, 226, 227, 230,
    303, 344, 345, 479, 481, 487,
    534, 668, 679
Medicago sp. 167

Melilotus albus 344
M. indicus 616
M. officinalis 344
Melilotus sp. 30

Onobrychis viciaefolia 601

Phaseolus sp. 492

Prosopis juliflora 258
P. juliflora var. velutina 112

Prosopis sp. 717

Robinia pseudoacacia 312, 613

Trifolium incarnatum 1, 344
T. pratense 30
T. repens 11
T. subterraneum 259
Trifolium sp. 48, 226, 227,
    279, 280, 345, 378, 405, 678,
    722, 747

Vigna sinensis 493

Lentibulariaceae
    Utricularia inflata 81

Liliaceae
    Asphodelus albus 368

    Hemerocallis fulva 262

    Uvularia sessilifolia 716

    Veratrum sp. 383

Limnanthaceae
    Limnanthes douglasii 23, 532,
        632
    Limnanthes sp. 466

Linaceae
    Linum mucronatum 356
    L. usitatissimum 589
    Linum sp. 792, 793

Loganiaceae
    Gelsemium sempervirens 276

208

Index

Lythraceae
  Cuphea llavea 778
  Cuphea sp. 465

Myrica sp. 387

Myrtaceae
  Myrciaria paraensis 90

Magnoliaceae
  Liriodendron tulipfera 218

  Magnolia sp. 744

Malpighiaceae
  Malpighia coccigera 321
  M. infestissima 321
  M. linearis 321
  M. shaferi 321
  M. suberosa 321

Malvaceae 664
  Anoda cristata 440

  Malva parviflora 440

Meliaceae
  Melia azerderach 182

  Trichilia sp. 211

Menispermaceae
  Cyclea peltata 382

Musaceae
  Musa cavendishi 249

Myricaceae
  Comptonia peregrina 716

  Myrica asplenifolia 292

Najadaceae
  Najas guadalupensis 81

Naucleaceae
  Cephalanthus occidentalis 411

Nelumbonaceae
  Nelumbo lutea 81, 411

Nymphaeaceae
  Nuphar adrena 81

  Nymphaea odorata 81, 89

Nyssaceae
  Nyssa sylvatica 381

Oleaceae
  Fraxinus americana 796
  F. pennsylvanica var. lanceolata
    218
  F. nigra 4
  Fraxinus sp. 6, 605

  Syringa vulgaris 157

Index

Index

Index

Index